Worried Sick?

The exaggerated fear of physical illness.

How to put physical symptoms into perspective.
How to avoid unnecessary worry.

By Fredric Neuman, M.D.

Simon & Brown
www.simonandbrown.com

ISBN-13: 978-0-9814843-4-1
ISBN-10: 0-9814843-4-4

Library of Congress Control Number: 2008928124
Library of Congress subject headings:
Health – Psychological
Compulsive Behavior
Health – Miscellanea

1.2

Author Online! To contact Dr. Neuman, please write to
info@simonandbrown.com

Worried Sick?

Table of Contents

Introduction: Why Worry?

No one likes to think of himself or herself as being emotionally disturbed or, worse, of having an emotional or mental illness of some sort. A person may readily admit to having gallstones or even a stomach ulcer yet hesitate to mention even to friends or to family a history of being clinically depressed. Some conditions, such as alcoholism, seem to be a kind of moral failure. Others, such as pseudocyesis, in which a woman imagines herself to be pregnant for 9 or 10 months, seem ridiculous, at least when they happen to other people. The exaggerated fear of physical illness, what may be called health anxiety, may strike some as falling into this category. The Woody Allen caricature of a hypochondriac is intended to make people laugh. From a certain point of view it is amusing to contemplate a vigorous young person anxiously taking his or her pulse and temperature every few minutes when the likelihood of being truly ill is vanishingly small. Health worriers, seeing themselves or their problems made fun of in this way, are especially not inclined to acknowledge those problems; and, consequently, they put themselves beyond help. I suspect this book may be bought as often by the families of health worriers as by the health worriers themselves.

Of course, whether someone is viewed with derision or with sympathy is a matter of perspective. Seeing a clown slip on a banana peel is funny as long as it seems clear he did not really hurt himself. Those men and women who have an inordinate fear of being sick *are* hurting. Having had this condition myself, I can testify to the awfulness of worrying about an illness which I knew was unlikely but which seemed threatening anyhow – and feeling foolish consequently for worrying unnecessarily. In a way, though, such a worry *is* funny. A man who thinks he may have had a heart attack because his left foot hurts is funny in a way, because his fear seems to us to be outlandish. I think it is permissible, even useful sometimes, to take note of someone's foible – or one's own foibles – and smile, as long as it is a sympathetic smile. Each of us has our own particular banana peel that we slip on over and over again in plain view of everybody. I try to be straightforward in this book and respectful. If some of the stories I tell are wryly amusing, it is not because I do not appreciate the real distress this condition causes.

Whether health anxiety should really be called an emotional illness in the first place is problematical. Psychiatrists are inclined to define any human weakness or quirk as an emotional disorder of some sort. If it were not an illness, they would not be reimbursed for treating it. Currently, there are two disorders listed in the Diagnostic and Statistical Manual (4th edition), which are closely related to health anxiety. These are hypochondriasis and somatization disorder. I give their definitions in Chapter One, and again more formally in the Index, but these descriptions are not very helpful. And there are other illnesses too, including panic disorder, obsessive-compulsive disorder and depression, which frequently cause physical symptoms and the fear of physical disease. I think it is more useful to describe health anxiety as simply an exaggerated fear of illness, this fear being an outgrowth of a set of mistaken ideas about the nature of physical illness, including its diagnosis and its treatment. It is more like a character trait, such as stinginess, than, let's say, schizophrenia, which is truly a disease in the sense that diabetes is a disease.

A Bad Idea

First, one may ask, how does someone come to believe false and frightening ideas about health, or about the world in general, for that matter, when everyday experience seems to everyone else to testify to a less frightening reality?

The scene: a rainy day in the Bronx, more than 50 years ago. The author, a fragile-appearing (by all accounts) 7 year old, has just come indoors.

The author's mother: Take off your rubbers, or you'll get sick.

The author: Sick? Why will I get sick?

The author's mother: Because if you wear your rubbers in the house, you'll catch cold.

The author: How come? How does my nose...how does any part of my body...even know I'm wearing rubbers outside my shoes?

The author's mother: Remember, I warned you.

Imagine endless variations on such a conversation repeated over and over again during childhood. What messages are communicated?

1. That health is easily damaged.
2. That slight deviations in ordinary matters, such as dress, predispose to illness.
3. That infectious disease is preventable.
4. That infectious diseases are always important enough to be prevented, if possible.

And what is the effect of hearing these messages, which become so much a part of growing up that they are like an invisible backdrop, taken for granted?

1. In my case, one becomes, first of all, skeptical. This is a useful turn of mind in a scientist (unfortunately, I am not a scientist), but annoying in someone who is around the house a lot.
2. Skeptical or not, one comes to accept the point of view of the parent, even if one rejects those particular superstitions and old wives' tales that the parent repeats. One does become worried about the precariousness of physical health.

After all, who speaks with more authority than one's own mother? Sometimes a traumatic event in childhood – a serious illness or the death of a family member – can by itself teach the same lessons. Even so, it is surprising, I think, that such ideas can survive into and sometimes throughout adulthood. I present an account in these pages of how health anxiety can suddenly appear in someone predisposed to it, let's say, by having over-protective parents. The related ideas that lead to health anxiety are varied. They include misconceptions about drugs and about laboratory tests, about illness per se, and about the way the human body functions when it is functioning normally. Treatment, of course, is directed at changing these ideas.

The Treatment of an Idea

Having been a director of psychiatric training for a number of years, I have watched from the other side of a one-way mirror therapists of all different theoretical persuasions conducting the therapy of all sorts of emotional disorders. Whether these practitioners describe themselves as psychoanalytically oriented or as believing in a cognitive or behavioral form of treatment, they tend, one way or another to work to a similar purpose. All of them argue one way or another against certain distortions in the way patients view the world.

"Just because your boss spoke harshly to you, it doesn't mean he plans on firing you."

"Just because your girlfriend danced with your friend, it doesn't mean she meant to humiliate you."

"Just because you walked into a sick room, it doesn't mean that you yourself will get sick."

Unfortunately, just listening to a therapist speak these truths, even a therapist whom the patient respects and trusts, is not convincing. Consequently, newer methods of treatment have grown up, especially in the management of panic disorder and of obsessive-compulsive disorder, conditions related to health anxiety; and these have been found useful in the treatment of health anxiety itself. They teach a lesson more successfully than the office-bound lectures of traditional psychotherapy. They are described in these chapters. To a considerable extent, they can be implemented without the continuing supervision of a therapist.

Health worriers are often very upset by routine interactions with their physicians. For that reason, I include a detailed account of the role of physicians, the process of diagnosis, and the meaning of laboratory results and other diagnostic procedures. I explain the various proper uses of medication. Whether or not to take medicine is always a matter of concern for health worriers. The placebo effect is described, including placebo side-effects. Implicit in much of what is discussed are strategies the health worrier can use to determine the likelihood of certain physical symptoms being due simply to the fact of being anxious and which others may reflect an underlying physical condition. There is a role for family members; and I offer some suggestions for them in a separate section.

Bad News

Every few years, it seems, a new disease appears to threaten us. A reunion of legionnaires is struck suddenly by a previously unknown, but potentially fatal, contagion. A number of children in Lyme, Connecticut develop a strange arthritis, which is found to be infectious in origin. AIDS, the so-called plague of the century, emerges in a number of countries simultaneously with consequences by now known to everyone. More recently, a number of previously healthy young people living in the Western part of the United States die suddenly after becoming infected with a hantavirus which they have caught somehow from the urine of a field mouse. Meanwhile, ancient diseases such as tuberculosis and malaria appear in a more virulent form. Unknown to those previous times are a whole range of poisons such as radon or asbestos or nitrates which invade our bodies insidiously, wreaking destruction. And familiar dangers turn out to be worse than we imagined. Cigarette smoke kills more people every year in the United States than were killed in all of its foreign wars put together. It appears that breathing, eating, and having sex all constitute threats to life. More threatening still are the largely degenerative conditions, such as cancer or cardiovascular diseases, that have in recent centuries killed the bulk of humankind, and that continue to do so now, as they will probably forever. Indeed, between one thing and another, those of us who avoid death by accident are killed by some disease eventually. We are not, most of us, prepared to accept this state of affairs lying down.

We do not graciously accept the idea of becoming sick, nor should we. Every few months we enter into a new strategy in the "war against cancer." Additional millions are spent by scientists to determine, once and for all, the underlying causes of heart disease, some of which, such as dietary overindulgence, have been known to everyone else's satisfaction for decades. The exact shape, chemically speaking, of the HIV virus is divined and published in the daily newspapers along with photographs so detailed and familiar that to the attentive reader the picture of this tiny organism budding out of a white cell is as recognizable as that of a chicken breaking out of an egg, with similar effect on the white cell as on the egg shell.

Good News

New tools for delving into the human body are trumpeted in the press. The CAT scan (computerized axial tomography) and the even more expensive MRI (magnetic resonance imaging) are surpassed in some ways by the PET scan (position emission tomography). It is possible now to portray the inside of the skull, a closed container, in successive cross-sections in marvelous exactitude so that the neurologist need no longer figure out what is going on in the brain, but can see directly. Similar technological advances have multiplied the diagnostic procedures that can be brought to bear by physicians on a particular medical problem. Someone determined to rule out a cryptic disease process can now spend considerable time and money on laboratory examinations that test much of the quirky ebb and flow of human physiology. Someone determined to ward off illness can engage in complicated strategies to do so, starting with the determination of a possible genetic vulnerability and ending with a beleaguered retreat from all the myriad toxins which are reputed to float through the air around us and also coat our foods. Finally, should these precautions fail, someone determined to search out a remedy for a particular illness has a whole range of drugs and procedures to draw upon. It is no wonder then that somebody who attends to the constant reporting in the media of disease and of the treatment of disease should become very focused on his or her own health, and overly worried.

Actually, the degree to which people worry about their health varies, with some people worrying too much and others not enough. Those that worry too much think that they are in greater danger than they really are, with unpleasant consequences that affect much of their lives; those that worry too little have trouble imagining that they might be truly ill and, therefore, do not take those measures that might prevent their getting still sicker. I would have trouble choosing, if I could, between these two extremes. Would it be better to wake up at intervals over a period of years with chest pain from indigestion and be so frightened of a heart attack that I end up each time going to a hospital emergency room; or would it be better to sail through life but fail to seek treatment for a real heart attack during those few hours when proper treatment can prevent cardiac damage? The fact is that many more people worry about their health unnecessarily than are unconcerned, for reasons that I will discuss later. It is for them that I have written this book. For it is possible to live effectively between these extremes.

Important Note: In order to make clear all the different Bad Ideas that underlie health anxiety, and to show just how debilitating this condition can be, I have drawn most of the case histories in this book from among the most troubled patients I have seen. Sometimes the case history is a composite of two or three such patients. The reader should understand, however, that very many people are affected to a lesser extent and sometimes only temporarily in the face of an obscure symptom or a transient illness. If the conditions are just right – or just wrong – perhaps anyone can be turned into a health worrier. These people too can find comfort by following the recommendations in this book. Sometimes, to offer a more balanced perspective, I describe cases that are less severe. I mark these N.S.B. (not so bad).

Chapter One: What is Health Anxiety?[1]

I am afraid that the image someone may have of a person who worries excessively about health is that of the ridiculous and somewhat pathetic hypochondriac that is often portrayed in the movies. It is true, of course, that nothing is more foolish than somebody else's irrational concerns. My fears, each person thinks, make more sense. Ambrose Bierce was speaking in a similar vein when he defined superstition as someone else's religion. But there is nothing ridiculous about being worried sick. Naturally, very few people are prepared to think of themselves as hypochondriacs. The implication is that there is nothing physically the matter with them, that their problem is "all in the head," and that their symptoms are imaginary. Indeed, the usual definition of hypochondriasis, which I give below, seems at first reading to say something similar.

The Diagnostic and Statistical Manual of Mental Disorders (4th Edition)

Published by the American Psychiatric Association.

Diagnostic criteria for hypochondriasis 300.7

A. The predominant disturbance is an unrealistic interpretation of physical signs or sensations as abnormal, leading to preoccupation with the fear or belief of having a serious disease.

B. Thorough physical evaluation does not support the diagnosis of any physical disorder that can account for the physical signs or sensations or for the individual's unrealistic interpretation of them.

C. The unrealistic fear or belief of having a disease persists despite medical reassurance and causes impairment in social or occupational functioning.

D. Not due to any other mental disorder such as Schizophrenia, Affective Disorder, or Somatization Disorder.

---

[1] See the scale at the end of this chapter. Someone who answers over half the questions <u>yes</u> should consider himself or herself a health worrier.

A related condition, somatization disorder, 300.10, is defined in these terms:

Diagnostic criteria for Somatization Disorder

A.   A history of many physical complaints beginning before age 30 years that occur over a period of several years and result in treatment being sought or significant impairment in social, occupational, or other important areas of functioning.

B.   Each of the following criteria must have been met, with individual symptoms occurring at any time during the course of the disturbance:

   (1)   *four pain symptoms:* a history of pain related to at least four different sites or functions (e.g., head, abdomen, back, joints, extremities, chest, rectum, during menstruation, during sexual intercourse, or during urination.)

   (2)   *two gastrointestinal symptoms:* a history of at least two gastrointestinal symptoms other than pain (e.g., nausea, bloating, vomiting other than during pregancy, diarrhea, or intolerance of several different foods.)

   (3)   *one sexual symptom:* a history of at least one sexual or reproductive symptom other than pain (e.g., sexual indifference, erectile or ejaculatory dysfunction, irregular menses, excessive menstrual bleeding, vomiting throughout pregnancy.)

      (1)   after appropriate investigation, the symptoms cannot be fully explained by a known medical condition or the direct effects of a substance (e.g., a drug of abuse, a medication)

      (2)   when there is a related general medical condition, the physical complaints or resulting

social or occupational impairment is in excess of what would be expected from the history, physical examination, or laboratory findings

C.   The symptoms cause clinically significant distress or impairment in social, occupational, or other important areas of functioning.

D.   The duration of the disturbance is at least 6 months.

These definitions, which have something of the aspect of a Chinese restaurant menu (take 3 symptoms from column A, 2 from column B...), leave out the greater number of people who worry unnecessarily and excessively about their health. Consider these three examples of what may be called health anxiety:

Adrienne is a middle-aged woman who reports that she has been worried about one thing or another most of her life. When she was a child, she was frightened by thunderstorms and by neighborhood dogs. Being left for a few hours with a baby-sitter made her inconsolable (and upset her mother too, who checked on her every hour by telephone). She cried throughout the first week of kindergarten and was so shy she had to be coaxed the next few years into attending the birthday parties of other children. Some of these problems became less evident with time only to return in somewhat different form in early adolescence when she developed what the school psychologist called a "full-blown school phobia." On school days she woke up with a stomachache which often cleared by mid-morning if she had been allowed to remain at home. If forced to attend school, she went to the nurse every day with headaches or a "strange, very jumpy" feeling. For a period of three weeks she refused to go to school at all. This problem too seemed to fade, perhaps because of the patient intervention of her guidance counselor.

Except for a slight, residual quirkiness – a nervousness about getting a good night's sleep and an inability to swallow pills – Adrienne grew up to be a self-confident, attractive woman with no discernible medical or psychological problems.

One evening, when Adrienne was 25 years old, she got stuck in traffic driving home from a friend's wedding. After a few moments of sitting quietly with her hands on the steering wheel of her automobile she suddenly became agitated, a feeling reminiscent of the attacks she used to have in school. A sense that something awful was happening swept over her. Her heart began to race, and she had trouble catching her breath. She experienced pain in her chest that seemed to radiate into her left shoulder, making her wonder if she was having a heart attack. She felt "spacey" and "unreal," and dizzy, not a spinning vertigo, but a kind of vague unsteadiness. She left the highway at the first exit and went to the nearest hospital emergency room. She was examined there and tested, including by electrocardiogram (EKG) and then released after being told there was nothing the matter with her, although she was told also to check with her regular physician the following day. He too could find no evidence of a medical illness. A week later she had a similar experience, and once again she went to a hospital. She was discharged with the same diagnosis – or lack of diagnosis – and with a prescription for a tranquilizer. These attacks were repeated with increasing frequency over the next few months until Adrienne was referred finally to a psychiatrist. By that time she was avoiding driving and also avoiding any other place where she felt trapped, such as restaurants or shopping centers.

The psychiatrist informed Adrienne that she had a panic disorder and suggested that she take anti-depressant drugs. However, she still had difficulty swallowing pills. Also, she was frightened by reports in the popular press of the potential side-effects of this class of drugs. Even taking one-eighth of a pill provoked a number of physical symptoms, including some that are seemingly opposite, such as sleepiness and insomnia, reactions that one would not expect to be caused simultaneously by the same medicine. Finally, because of the severity of these presumed side-effects, and because Adrienne thought they might worsen and become truly dangerous to her, she refused to take these drugs or any other psychoactive medication, save only the minor tranquilizers which she was on already. Although these were not helping her, she had perversely become dependent on them and was unable or unwilling to go anywhere without taking them beforehand.

Although Adrienne understood quite well that she was emotionally upset, even to an unwarranted degree, she was convinced nevertheless that she was suffering also from some obscure and possibly deadly medical disease that her doctor was missing. As time went on she went from doctor to doctor, encouraging them to perform any and every test that might conceivably uncover that hidden ailment. Her nagging tended to alienate even those among her physicians who were sympathetic to her distress – and not all of them were. They regarded her as clinging. She saw them as unresponsive and uninterested.

Adrienne's condition did not improve much over the succeeding months and years. Her panic attacks became less frequent, but she was still afraid of them. She continued to worry that she might have an underlying heart condition, despite her doctors' reassurance that she was the wrong age and the wrong sex and had no other risk factors. Nor were her concerns limited to heart disease. As soon as she woke up every morning she checked her breathing "to make sure I'm still alive," she commented wryly. Then she took her pulse to see if her heart was skipping a beat as it did sometimes. When she got out of bed, finally, she was careful to test her balance to see if she got that "weird, dizzy" feeling, which she usually did or that "spacey" feeling which she got sometimes when she had not eaten for a while, and which she had been told by one doctor was due to low blood pressure and by another was due to low blood sugar.

On those uncommon occasions when she developed an upper respiratory infection or a gastroenteritis, she worried that she had a more serious condition. She took her temperature and pulse eight or nine times a day and worried if there was too much of a spread between the highest readings and the lowest. Although she had little knowledge about the factors that might affect her heart rate, she had the idea that an elevated heart rate was unhealthy if it went on too long. Headaches led her to think that she might have a brain tumor. She examined her eyes to see if they had become reddened and her tongue to see if it had developed a coating. Any variation from what she conceived to be normal frightened her. She was afraid also that without medical intervention any medical condition she developed would get worse rather than better. Consequently, she was always alert to the first sign of any such condition.

This preoccupation waxed and waned depending on circumstances, including matters of such little relevance to Adrienne's health as reports in the press of other people's illnesses. At her best she was only mildly distracted and discomforted by these thoughts. At her worst she was anxious all day long and could think of little else.

*　　*　　*

Although Adrienne's mother was said to be a "worrier," Robert's parents, as far as he could remember, were calm, at least about matters of health. His father might have been said to be eccentric, perhaps, always straightening photographs and aligning his shoes just so in his closet; but he was otherwise unremarkable. Unfortunately, when Robert was 10, his father developed the first signs of the wasting disease that finally killed him five years later. Despite this traumatic experience Robert grew up seemingly emotionally mature and stable. He became a lawyer and was successful. Like his father, he too had an exaggerated need for orderliness, especially in matters of dress. He also required a precise amount of sleep and ate only healthy foods prepared in a certain way; but in his mind being well-organized and circumspect was admirable and accounted in no small measure for his professional success.

When Bob was 22, he developed a minor illness which was thought to be viral but which lingered in the form of a low-grade fever for months. During this time a close friend died from Hodgkin's disease, a form of lymphatic cancer. When it became apparent that no doctor was able to say exactly what illness Bob was suffering from, he began to think that possibly he had some unusual form of cancer that the doctors were missing. He palpated his lymph nodes every few minutes, wondering if they were swelling. Probably as the result of his prodding, one lymph node became so inflamed it had to be removed surgically. The ensuing few days, when he had to wait for the pathological report on the lymph node, were especially trying. He lost his appetite and was unable to sleep; and this disturbance of his daily routine threatened, he thought, to worsen whatever illness he had. He also began to attend abnormally to other aspects of bodily functioning. He examined his stools and worried if they varied from what seemed to him to be normal. His urine, he noticed, sometimes became dark; and he reported this to his current physician who was said to be an expert on obscure diseases. A considerable battery of tests was performed, a few of which were reported back out of the range of normal, precipitating still other tests. For reasons that no one was able to explain later on, an MRI was ordered. However, the enclosed cavity of the MRI was too threatening, and Bob refused the test at the last moment.

In time, Bob's fever disappeared; but he did not feel well. He was angry at the inability of his various doctors to explain why he had become ill, why he developed the particular symptoms he had, and why he had them at that particular period of his life, when he had never had them before. He also never found out why his abnormal laboratory tests had been abnormal. More important, he suspected he was still ill. Although he had had sexual intercourse with no one but his wife in the previous seven years, he worried that somehow he might have contracted AIDS. He also began to worry about germs in general. He would not swim in a public pool or drink from someone else's glass for fear of germs. His finicky attitude towards food now became so exaggerated he had trouble eating enough to maintain his weight. Foods that touched, or may have touched, dirty utensils became inedible. He washed his hands repetitively and at such length that they became raw. Ultimately, all areas of his life were compromised by this pathological fastidiousness.

Eventually, Bob's emotional symptoms were improved considerably on a drug regimen, which included anti-depressants and tranquilizers. However, he was never entirely free of worries about his health. A transient fever set him worrying again about AIDS. Negative tests for AIDS, repeated a number of times, did not reassure him. He imagined himself wasting away in bed, helpless, his family staring at him with that mixture of dismay and disapproval that AIDS often engenders. He was always careful not to exert himself too much, or eat or sleep too much, or too little. A routine physical examination made him anxious for a week before and for days after until all the tests were reported back normal. Any feeling of unsteadiness, or any other vague feeling, made him think he was sick; and any real sickness made him think he might be deathly ill. And, this was his condition whether he was on medication or not.

*　　*　　*

Emma was a "worry-wart" as far back as she could remember; but she did not remember worrying about health any more than she worried about getting good grades or about the danger of driving through unsafe neighborhoods. She used to worry about her kid sister being left with a babysitter. However, when she was 17 she was terribly upset by the sudden illness of a friend who had a stroke, from which the woman luckily made a full recovery. Prior to the stroke, the young woman had complained to Emma of dizziness and a stomachache, symptoms almost certainly not connected to the cause of her stroke. Nevertheless, seemingly from that point on,

Emma developed headaches and symptoms of what was described variously as acid indigestion or hiatus hernia. Subsequently, after considerable medical work-up, an additional diagnosis was made of irritable bowel syndrome. These were the first of a number of ill-defined conditions attributed to Emma more or less casually by one physician or another over the years. When she developed pain and vague tenderness in different muscle groups, she was told she had fibromyalgia. Someone else suggested chronic pain syndrome. When she felt especially tired after a lingering sinusitis, she was told she had developed chronic fatigue syndrome. She had a runny nose and a post-nasal drip and was told by a doctor said to be expert in chemical sensitivities that she had a chemical sensitivity syndrome. He instructed her further to avoid all food additives and not to handle newsprint. Along the way she was also told she had mitral valve prolapse and hypoglycemia, but not to worry about them. There were other illnesses that came up from time to time as possibilities, at least in Emma's mind, as she questioned her doctors in an attempt to figure out what was always going wrong with her health. A partial list of these included migraine, peptic ulcer, lumbar disc rupture, endometriosis, and onychomycosis, which is fungal infection of the toe nails. Having become frantic contemplating these possibilities, she was told also that she had generalized anxiety disorder (GAD). 300.02

Like any other preoccupation, Emma's concerns about her health came and went depending on circumstances. When she was due for a routine physical examination or test, such as a PAP smear, the thought of it intruded at intervals days ahead of time into her mind, no matter what else she was doing. Often, because she was anxious, she postponed or neglected medical visits or procedures. The unwelcome thoughts that distressed her were hard for her to describe, and painful. One awful scene she imagined was the doctor looking somberly at her and telling her, "I'm sorry, but you have cervical cancer." Although typically she avoided routine medical visits, when she was sick, even slightly, she was immediately in the doctor's office and frequently on the telephone soon afterward to make sure she understood what the doctor had said – and, to make sure he had understood what she had told him. Often she felt that he had not been attentive to her and had not been forthcoming in his explanation of her problem.

This state of affairs, which is not unusual for health worriers, persisted for years. Emma took a turn for the worse, however, when she became a mother. Soon thereafter, her fears began to center on cancer, and breast cancer in particular. She developed the habit of examining her breasts before going out in the evening with her husband "to make sure I'm okay, so I can relax." More often than not, however, she found some irregularity or thickening that suggested to her the presence of a lump; and the evening would be ruined. A particular thought troubled her especially. She imagined the awful things likely to happen to her children <u>after</u> she died of cancer. She thought of their being helpless and alone at all the critical times of their lives. And, she thought of herself not being able to see them graduate from school or get married. Inevitably, whenever her children became ill, Emma would imagine them sicker than they really were, despite the reassurance of her pediatrician. Once she ventured to ask him if her daughter, who was running a fever, might be suffering from muscular dystrophy, a devastating disease she had recently heard described on television. The description, by the way, suggested no resemblance to her daughter's illness. Had she been able to listen properly, she would have been reassured by the program rather than frightened by it. At other times she stayed up all night listening to her daughter cough and conjuring up visions of other terrible diseases.

To this point in her life, Emma had not sought psychiatric treatment because neither she nor the people around her considered her to be emotionally ill. She was regarded simply as someone who worried too much about matters of health.

*   *   *

None of these three people entirely satisfied the strict criteria which the American Psychiatric Association has set out in its definitions of hypochondriasis or somatization disorder. Adrienne suffered from a panic disorder, which, for purposes of diagnosis at least, supersedes the diagnosis of hypochondriasis. Robert's severe depression is an affective disorder, which would also take precedence over consideration of his health worries, even though those concerns were a principal part of his distress. His symptoms at various times would have also required the diagnosis of obsessive-compulsive disorder. Emma had been diagnosed as generalized anxiety disorder. All three at one point in their lives at least had physical illnesses that seemed to account for their physical symptoms. Although all three were socially impaired at some point by their health worries, at other times these worries subsided into a psychological background which was largely invisible to others except, perhaps, to their families.

The following story, which is my own, is an example of someone less affected that the three people described above. My condition, also, could not have been squeezed comfortably into the official definitions for hypochondriasis or somatization disorder. I do not think my problem ever rose to the level of social or occupational impairment, but it certainly caused me considerable and unnecessary distress.

Memory is unreliable; and I imagine mine is no better than anyone else's. I would not want anyone to judge my parents by what I remember of them, not that they would have sought my approval particularly. They had their own opinions, which they held to strongly. Some of their ideas may have been sensible. In any case, they meant well. Also, I am generally disinclined to blame parents, mine or anyone else's, for their children's problems. There is a long, ignoble tradition of blaming parents, mothers in particular, for their children's emotional illnesses, including, for example, schizophrenia and childhood autism, both of which are known now to be caused bio-logically for the most part. This is not to say, of course, that parents do not have considerable influence over their children's future lives. Plainly they do. Much of what we believe we have learned from them. Some of these ideas impact our lives in unhealthy ways. But we do not stop learning when we become adults. Books such as this one are dedicated to the principle that people can change and become better, and, certainly, less troubled. In that sense, of course, we are responsible for ourselves, no matter what our childhood was like.

In many ways, I had a favored childhood. I was the center of attention, at least my mother's attention. But my parents were fright-ened people. Mostly, it seemed to me, they worried about me. They worried about my getting too little sleep, too much sun, not enough rest and just the right amount of food – and the right kind of food. Hot dogs and other stadium foods were off-limits. Cod liver oil was good; and I can taste it still. Fresh air was good, as long as you were dressed warmly, but sleeping in a draft was likely to cause illness, including paralysis of the facial muscles. For that matter, creasing up your forehead, I was told, would lead to permanent wrinkles. Air conditioning could make you sick, also cold fluids, especially if you drank them when you were hot and thirsty. All alcoholic beverages were bad and even ritual wine was doled out in glasses so small they might have been taken from a set of dollhouse furniture. Reading in a car or in dim light hurt your eyes. Loud music hurt your ears. Ill-fitting shoes hurt your feet. I grew up in a world fraught with danger, but dangers that could be avoided if you were careful. My father prevented my developing tooth problems, he boasted to me years later, by tying down my thumbs <u>before</u> I could learn to suck on them!

As I grew somewhat older, I was warned against getting too close to electrical outlets in order to avoid sparks, and too close to the curb in case a car drove up on the sidewalk. I was especially warned against approaching closer than six feet to the chest-high wall which enclosed the roof of our apartment building where we spent most of our summers. After all, I was slight, and occasional strong breezes below across the roof. I was given eye exercises to improve my nearsightedness. I was taken to the eye doctor regularly to remove waxy build-up from my eyelid. He treated what I learned later was an allergic conjunctivitis with a silver-nitrate cauterization, a painful and ineffective procedure. My hair was combed with a fine-tooth comb to prevent something or other, probably lice. Naturally, I had to stay away from the foods I was allergic to, or was supposed to be allergic to. I came across a list of these a few years ago. Thirty-seven food were listed, including cold water!

There were other dangers. My father drove carefully on the painted line in the middle of the road in order to avoid sideswiping parked cars. He had no car radio because in his opinion you could not drive safely and listen to music at the same time. He drove slowly and <u>never</u> in my experience passed another car unless it was disabled. I used to stare disconsolately through the back window at the long line of cars that stretched behind us. I was taught how to avoid being struck by lightning (stay away from appliances and open windows) and told never to swim right after eating. This was useless advice since I was never permitted near a body of water larger than that in a bathtub; and I was warned to be careful in there too. Neither of my parents could swim and yet both had almost drowned, they told me. Between one thing and another, I did not myself learn to swim until I was 17 or learn how to drive an automobile until I was 28. I was not allowed to roller-skate or bicycle because I might injure my hands. I was walked to the bus up to a relatively advanced age to prevent my getting mugged. I was not the only one thought to be fragile. I was advised not to aggravate my father any further because he had an enlarged heart. There was no evidence of an enlarged heart when he died 50 years later at the age of 89. Even mechanical devices were inclined to falter. I was told not to turn the station dial on the radio back and forth too much lest the radio break.

I do not remember as a kid worrying much myself, but I must have complained about physical symptoms of one sort or another because I remember being frequently in doctors' offices.

"Those are hunger pains, only <u>hunger</u> pains," I remember one doctor saying, trying unsuccessfully to reassure my mother about me.

"I know he hears a tone when he's in a quiet room. That's <u>normal</u>," said another doctor.

Inevitably, since I went from one doctor to another, I was told from time to time that I had a condition which, in fact, I did not have, an experience that would recur many times subsequently. For example, I developed postural hypotension, which is the benign tendency, especially among adolescents, for blood pressure to drop a little when standing up. Most people do not notice the woozy feeling they get under those circumstances – or, at least, they do not complain of it. On the other hand, when I had this minor symptom, my mother and I found our way to a number of doctors. We were told first that I had hypothyroidism, and then a year later by another physician that I suffered from hypoglycemia. It's lucky I did not have these conditions since the treatments that were recommended to me, I now know, were wrong. Along the way, I had some real illnesses, including generalized vaccinia, a rare and often fatal complication of an ordinary smallpox vaccination; and these too may have helped to provoke the exaggerated tendency to worry about my health that I noticed first in myself about the time I began to attend college.

I think I was at first simply inclined to pay attention to aspects of bodily function that seemed to be below everyone else's notice. My vision would blur unpredictably. Shooting pains came and went. Joints made interesting crepitant sounds. I discovered bumps here and there and moles in graduated sizes. I was more bemused than worried.

One day, however, when sitting in class, I had a sudden sense

14

of something going terribly wrong. My heart started to pound, and I could not catch my breath. I felt wobbly and off-balance. I thought I could not hear. Certainly, I could not pay attention; and the feelings seemed to worsen every moment. Striking though these physical symptoms were, more distracting still was an awful feeling that I was about to lose control of myself – scream, or in some other way embarrass myself. I thought I was going crazy. I felt better an hour later, but similar attacks recurred every few days.

A nervous search through the psychological literature suggested that I was suffering what was then called anxiety attacks, and now called panic disorder. In the wake of these episodes I developed an agoraphobia, which is essentially the fear of being trapped somewhere, such as in a classroom, from where it is difficult to escape quickly. I need not, for purposes of this book, describe how I eventually got better. There did come a time when I no longer had panic attacks and was not phobic. Unfortunately, the worries I had about my health became more exaggerated and, judging from the teasing of friends and family, more ridiculous. These problems improved and then worsened again off and on for a period of years depending on circumstances. During that period, when things were at their worst, I noticed that whatever particular worries I had at that moment, certain habits of mind were always there:

1. A tendency when I got sick to consider the most serious illness I might have rather than the most common and benign. Later on, when I knew the illness I was worrying about was unlikely, I worried about it anyway.

2. The thought that when I was sick I needed to go to a doctor in order to get better. Growing up in the city, I thought nature itself would break down without human beings to manage it. It came as a revelation when I moved to suburbia to discover that squirrels could survive on their own without anyone feeding them peanuts. In other words, I had the vague idea that medical problems naturally got worse rather than better. Not infrequently, I

went to see a doctor before I had developed symptoms characteristic enough to make a diagnosis.

3. Having concluded that I had not much reason to worry, whatever
   worry I was trying to put aside would nevertheless suddenly
   spring to mind throughout the day. Particular images, such as
   being told that a lab result was positive, or lying helpless in a hospital bed, haunted me.

4. A sensitivity to other people's medical catastrophes. A friend who
   got sick in some striking way would set me thinking willy-nilly of
   myself and my own symptoms, sometimes setting me to examine
   my body compulsively. Sometimes I noticed an irregularity of
   some sort, a bump or an asymmetry, which, no doubt, I had
   always had but had never noticed before. At other times I tested
   my balance to make sure I had not become off-balance somehow.

5. A tendency to worry similarly about other people close to me.
   Years later, when I became a parent, the exaggerated concerns I
   had about my own health merged with similar preoccupations
   about my children's well-being. Although I was a physician, I
   tended to worry that they might be sicker than they really were.
   Often, I slept on the floor of their rooms when they had a febrile
   illness.

   Finally, I noticed eventually that I had a tendency to develop
physical symptoms, such as headaches or cramps, when I was under
certain kinds of stress. However, knowing this did not stop me from
wondering on those occasions whether those symptoms might be
caused, this time, by an underlying medical illness.

   If I had been examined by a psychiatrist, I might have been
diagnosed as having a number of different illnesses, or none,
depending on which concerns I had currently; and these varied
sometimes from week to week.

   Emotional disorders, like every other illness, are defined by nature, not by man. Psychiatrists, nevertheless, maintain a peculiar conceit, which allows them to define and then redefine emotional illnesses every few years.

Homosexuality, for example, was voted out a few years ago by a small majority vote and is now normal. When borderline mental retardation was abandoned as a diagnostic category a few years later, the greater number of people previously regarded as mentally retarded were "cured" at a single stroke. In that tradition, I would like to suggest that this condition too should be reconsidered. I think health anxiety should be defined in terms of those particular ideas that are central to the disorder, and by those behaviors that grow directly out of those ideas. Some of these are mentioned in the previous pages. Health anxiety is marked by:

1. Persistent, even obsessional worries about being sick, those concerns existing out of proportion to any real symptoms or real illness that the person may have. <u>Judging by that standard alone, it is apparent that many people, even most people, have had this problem at some point in their lives</u>.

2. The tendency to attribute symptoms to an obscure but <u>profound</u>, perhaps fatal, illness. There may be a tendency to focus on one particular illness over others just as serious. Fears of AIDS, cancer, or an impending heart attack are especially common.

3. Repeated compulsive acts of self-monitoring for the presence of symptoms, usually supplying no substantive information. Taking one's pulse or temperature are examples.

4. The need for continual although ineffective reassurance from families and doctors. (Many doctors, usually). The search for an elusive certainty by performing more and more tests.

5. An ambivalent (dependent-demanding-resentful) relationship with those doctors.

6. A similarly contradictory attitude toward drugs. The health worrier starts with the idea that all drugs are more potent than they really are – with two consequences:

a. He or she is disinclined to take any prescribed medication because of the fear of possible side-effects, sometimes to the point of refusing them absolutely.

b. Once having begun on drugs, he or she is afraid to give them up. Tranquilizers, in particular, come to seem necessary in order to get through the day safely or in order to fall asleep successfully.

People who worry about their health may have other worries too. Therefore:

7. A correlation exists with other emotional disorders so that the health worrier may at various times fulfill the diagnostic criteria for phobias or obsessive-compulsive disorder. These conditions too can be defined largely by the particular fears of the individual, in the case of phobias by fears of traveling, for instance, or fear of loss of self-control; in the case of obsessive-compulsive disorder, the fear of contamination among other fears. Depression is commonly related to health anxiety, sometimes as a cause, sometimes as an effect. The overlap of these conditions is important and has implications for treatment. More of this later.

When someone becomes distressed in all these ways, it is usually obvious to everyone - although sometimes last to the affected person himself - that his or her reaction to illness or to the possibility of being ill is exaggerated and unwarranted. That person is suffering from an <u>emotional</u> problem, <u>whether or not</u> he or she is physically ill too. When the condition is less severe, however, when fewer of these core elements are present, it becomes possible to think that however upset the person may be, perhaps it is not out of proportion to the perceived threat. "Given these particular symptoms," one may think, "and judging from what the doctor said, or didn't say, or what the laboratory test said, or didn't say, wouldn't <u>anyone</u> worry?" It is precisely the character of an irrational fear that it appears reasonable to the person having it; and, if that person is bright enough, he or she can be convincing to family and to others and sometimes even to doctors! Besides, no one likes to be identified as a hypochondriac, not just because the image conjured up is slightly ridiculous, but because the health worrier wants his or her physical symptoms to be taken seriously. If he has an irregular heart beat, he does not want the doctor to dismiss it ahead of time as just one more psychosomatic complaint. If she can feel another lump in her breast, she wants this one examined carefully even if all the others vanished as soon as the doctor looked for them. For this reason, some patients who may be seeing a psychiatrist refuse to say so when they visit their regular doctor. No one wants to think - or wants others to think - that physical symptoms are simply imaginary. And, indeed, the fact is, they are not. But sooner or later health worriers come to understand that, however they manage to appear to others, they do worry more than they should. That is the simple standard someone should use to decide whether or not he or she has something that might reasonably be called health anxiety.

This book offers a treatment program for those who worry too much about their health, and, beyond that, teaches precepts that have been found in other contexts to dissipate other sorts of irrational fears. Following it leads to a more realistic and more comfortable way of living.

It might be useful to draw a contrast between those case histories mentioned above and that of another man who reacted differently to the threat of physical illness:

I cannot report reliably on Sanford's childhood since he is not introspective and says he remembers little of this period of his life. However, a principal event, surely, was the sudden death of his father when he was eleven. The loss of a parent at such a time is known to predispose to depression, but such proved not to be the case this time. Instead, Sanford became independent and, very quickly, self-assured, even, to some extent, cocky. When he graduated college he started his own business with very little capital and then talked a bank into giving him a big loan.

One day Sanford noticed his heart was beating irregularly. There were skipped beats, extra thumping beats, and occasional runs of fast beats. There was an interesting musical quality to the arrhythmia, Sanford thought. He wondered vaguely just when this disturbance started but figured it would probably go away in a few days "the same way it came." He did not bother to mention the problem to his wife. A few weeks later it had not yet gone away and, consequently, he found his way to the nearest doctor, who happened to have an office around the corner. The doctor took an EKG, which she described as "curious." She wanted to show it to a cardiologist, she said, before deciding how to proceed further.

That evening, when Sanford called to find out what the cardiologist had said, she told him:

"Well, there are a lot of PVCs in the EKG record; but it probably means nothing".

Sanford: "Is it okay to play racquetball tonight"

Doctor: "Sure. The cardiologist said you can do anything you would ordinarily do."

Sanford played racquetball that night with his usual competitive fervor. His arrhythmia disappeared some time later. He could not have said exactly when.

What is worth noting in Sanford's response to his heart arrhythmia?

1. Although he experienced a disturbance of function in a vital organ (the heart), he did not immediately suspect that he was sick. At no point did he consider the possibility that he was *seriously* sick. When he first got palpitations, he waited to see a doctor on the assumption that the condition would probably go away by itself.

2. When he did go to a doctor, it was not with the expectation that the doctor would make his heart irregularity disappear, possibly

with medication, or even that the doctor would be able to tell him why he had developed this symptom in the first place. It was with the idea that the doctor would instruct him on what if anything needed to be done. Laying out a plan of this sort is what doctors are trained to do.

3. Since Sanford had been reassured by his doctor, he felt secure engaging in strenuous exercise. He did not think it necessary to be reassured the next day because his heart irregularity was slightly different or because he had a headache too - or because he had eaten a fatty meal, or slept poorly, or skipped his tranquilizer, or taken an extra one inadvertently, or for any other reason.

Summing up Sanford's attitude: it reflected an expectation that he was not likely to become ill and certainly not dangerously ill. In other words, he was not a health worker. Sanford did not do so well in every area of his life. His unshakable aplomb prevented him sometimes from anticipating untoward events, which he should have been able to foresee. He did not worry sometimes when he should have done so, with unfortunate consequences in his business and romantic life. It should be noted, however, that an optimistic point of view usually leads to success in these areas.

Health worriers, on the other hand, have a number of ideas about illness and about their bodies that sum to the opposite conclusion: they expect to get seriously ill. They have other ideas also that tend to make them miserable.

Bad Ideas with a Capital B

All the anxiety disorders can be defined in terms of certain dysfunctional ideas. People afflicted with these conditions have incorrect ideas about themselves or about the world. I call these ideas "Bad Ideas with a capital B" because often these ideas determine, even define, the lives of those who hold them. These notions may not be acknowledged consciously or explicitly, but someone looking at the behavior of a neurotic person would conclude that they were implicit in that person's statements or in the way they interacted with the people around them. "Bad Ideas" are inaccurate and self-defeating, and, literally, worrisome. They also often have the character of being a self-fulfilling prophecy. Someone who has learned in childhood to be suspicious of the motives of other people will in adulthood behave in a guarded and sometimes hostile manner which may elicit just the sort of unpleasant behavior from others that they expect – serving to confirm those ideas. Consider these other examples of Bad Ideas:

A phobia is an exaggerated fear of a place, a thing, or a set of circumstances. Among the specific phobias that people suffer are a fear of animals or insects, lightning, heights and so on. Agoraphobia, of which claustrophobia is one variant, is a fear of being trapped in certain situations where the phobic feels he or she might suddenly get panicky and be unable to escape. Such places typically include trains or airplanes, elevators, shopping centers, theaters, tunnels and bridges and the like. A closely related condition is social phobia, which includes a fear of public speaking and elaborate social events such as weddings. Phobic persons typically share these views among others:

About the world: The world is a dangerous place. The farther away you get from home the more danger you are in. It is safer to be with someone than by yourself. Family members are safest of all. Strangers are likely to be unsympathetic rather than helpful.

About themselves: Feelings can get out of control, causing people to engage in embarrassing or dangerous behavior such as screaming or driving off a bridge. Health is precarious. Drugs are frightening. Note the overlap with health anxiety.

These ideas, which in this formulation might seem overstated to the average phobic person, are a largely unconscious bias to think certain thoughts, feel a certain way, and engage in certain behaviors. The result is recognizable as what we mean by a phobia.

Obsessive-compulsive disorder is a condition in which people engage in ritual warding-off behaviors such as repetitive, sometimes constant, hand washing. Unwanted, anxiety-provoking thoughts intrude into consciousness. Often these concern invisible dangers such as germs or other contaminants. The compulsive person repeatedly checks to see if the stove is turned off or the front door is locked. The hallmark of obsessive-compulsive disorder is doubt and the search for an unobtainable certainty by endlessly counting and checking. The Bad Ideas that drive obsessive-compulsives are visible moving not far below the surface of their lives. Like the phobic, they too believe the world is a dangerous place, but filled in particular with invisible dangers. Compulsive persons overvalue cleanliness and symmetry. They believe, unlike certain Christians, in the perfectibility of human behavior and in the avoidability of risk if one is careful enough.

The anxiety disorders, all of them, reflect one particular over-riding view of life: it is that the world is frightening. This view is a caricature and, therefore, false. It is misleading; and someone who lives strictly by such a tenet may very well be considered emotionally ill.

How is it possible, then, one might wonder, for such a set of stereotyped behaviors and attitudes to evolve? And why would such a set of dysfunctional and self-defeating ideas persist?

If I close my eyes, I can imagine a primitive society, way back when, during a period of our collective past, which must have lasted throughout the greater part of our history. I see a small tribe managing a precarious existence in a place where the possibility of sudden catastrophe was always present, when a bite from a small animal or a broken leg surely meant death, and when strangers from other tribes were likely to prove hostile. Perched on a lookout, on top the entrance to a cave, is a man, arms akimbo (I'm not sure I've got this entirely right) staring at a nearby line of trees to see if his sons are back from hunting. At the same time he searches for signs of a storm, for bears, and for the subtle movement of snakes that a less vigilant person might not notice. He is the tribal phobic. His wife is below at the entrance to the cave tending to the fire, checking repeatedly to make sure that it burns still and her baby does not reach for a stray ember. In between she ventures into the recesses of the cave, where her husband does not feel comfortable, to remove some food remains before they attract rats. She is the tribal obsessive-compulsive. Meanwhile, her elderly sister is nearby chewing thoughtfully on a new herb she has collected. Is it bitter? Has it made her tongue hairy? Or her bowels to rise? Hers is the role of nurse/physician. She is the tribal hypochondriac.

Each of these archetypal worriers served an important function for their community. Perhaps the race would not have survived had not someone like them been watching out for the very real dangers of those times.

But the world is different now. We have little to fear from wild beasts or from straying too far from home, and less now to fear from physical illness. People live now consistently longer than ever before. Why - and, more important, how - do such systematic fears develop? How do particular individuals in this day and age learn to be afraid and continue to be afraid in the absence of real danger? This question is part of a still larger issue. How do we maintain throughout life the prejudices we learn in childhood? For example, how can a woman live into middle-age and think that all men are sadists? How can a man who has had considerable work experience feel that all bosses are exploitative and all workers derelict? As in the example of the suspicious man described previously, these are self-confirming ideas. A woman who thinks men are interested in women primarily for sex is likely to behave in ways, either defensively or seductively, that cause them to react in sexual terms. She is also likely to notice those times especially and to remember them selectively, both of which serve to confirm her opinion. It is for this reason that psychotherapists have trouble portraying the world positively to emotionally disturbed persons. That view conflicts with a lifetime of their own experience.

*   *   *

More than the other people I have described so far, Rebecca's symptoms were almost entirely that of health anxiety. She had no complaints suggesting obsessive-compulsive disorder or an agoraphobia. She had no history of panic attacks; and she never developed symptoms suggesting a clinical depression. Her problems began, at the age of 18, it seemed to her, when she was told she had mitral valve prolapse, a common and minor irregularity of the heart, of no more significance, in fact, her cardiologist added, than having a receding chin. Nevertheless, from that time on, Rebecca had a sensitivity to her heart. She noticed extra beats or fast beats. She worried if her pulse accelerated "too much" when she climbed stairs or became emotionally upset. Consequently, she avoided "stress" whenever she could, and also physical exercise. Consequently, she became fat. As she got older, she suffered chronically from a variety of pains, including back pain, and other physical problems, especially cramps and loose stools. These were a distraction every day, and sometimes worse, interfering with work and any other activity that took place at a distance from a bathroom. Three different barium enemas revealed no pathology in her colon. Three barium enemas represent a considerable amount of radiation for a woman of childbearing age. When she became more seriously ill, as she did once with a peptic ulcer, she became so anxious she needed tranquilizers in order to sleep.

These symptoms became abruptly worse when she required a D and C, an ordinarily minor surgical procedure for excessive menstrual bleeding. She came out of anesthesia in severe pain. When she told the medical staff repeatedly that there was "something going wrong," they patted her on the head and reassured her that "everything was fine." A few minutes later, when she was being rushed back into the operating room and just before sinking into unconsciousness, she heard the distraught doctor telling a nurse,

"Hurry, we're losing her." It turned out she was hemorrhaging. She survived this medical emergency without physical sequelae; but her health anxiety worsened.

A particular set of related ideas contributed to her overall anxiety about her health. She had a mistaken understanding about the nature of physical illness, about her own particular vulnerability to illness, about the meaning of certain laboratory results, about the effect of drugs, and about the likelihood of developing a fatal disease. And she had other such notions. She was even mistaken in how she pictured the process of dying itself. She developed these ideas because of the circumstances of her life.

Just two among these ideas can be singled out to illustrate how ordinary life experiences can sustain a false view of the world. She believed, among other things:

Bad Idea #1: That she was more likely to get sick than other people. No matter how rare a disease was, she felt-with her luck-she would get it.

Bad Idea #2: That doctors were not reliable. In particular, she felt that doctors were not likely to take her physical complaints seriously, but were inclined to dismiss them as "emotional" or even imaginary.

Learning a Bad idea. Parents have great influence, which is why most people share the religious views and, to a lesser extent, the political views of their parents.

Bad Idea # 1: There was no mystery in how Rebecca came to believe she was more sickly than other children: Her mother told her so. "If somebody else gets a cold, you're likely to get pneumonia," she said, dragging her off to one doctor or another. Rebecca was not allowed in the company of sick children, lest she too become sick. When one case of equine encephalitis was reported in the local newspaper, Rebecca was told to stay indoors to avoid mosquitoes. The same message was implicit in other actions her mother took, for example, giving her extra vitamin C if she sneezed – or if she had been in the company of someone who sneezed!

Bad Idea #2: When Rebecca was small, she was often taken from one doctor's office one day to another the next. Her mother would ask the doctor "Are you sure?" or "How do you know it isn't leukemia?" The underlying suggestion, heard only dimly, perhaps, by Rebecca, but repeatedly, was that doctors had to be reminded to be diligent.

Reinforcing a Bad Idea. Bad ideas are maintained and confirmed by certain systematic errors of thinking, some of which are given below.

A. Selective Attention: Rebecca, like everyone else, was inclined to notice certain things more than others.

Bad Idea #1: Put simply, Rebecca noticed every time she got sick. She did not notice those times when she had been exposed to someone else's illness and did not get sick. She especially noticed those times when she was very sick. Since other people, when they were very sick, were home in bed and out of view, Rebecca tended to believe that she got sicker than other people, and more frequently. Instead of simply getting ill, like everyone does from time to time for no particular reason, she attributed her illnesses to a basic physical weakness.

Bad Idea #2: Occasionally, the doctors whom Rebecca visited for her various ailments turned out to be wrong, that is, they might say to her something on the order of "I think you may have X" when it turned out a few weeks later she really had Y. These times were disquieting to her despite the fact that there was often no difference in treatment for X and Y and despite the fact that she invariably got better anyway. She did not notice the far greater number of times the doctors were right. Also, she was inclined to interpret their hesitation to order tests for far-out diseases as carelessness or indifference.

B. <u>Distorted Observation</u> Inclined to a particular belief, Rebecca tended to consider events in her life in terms of that belief. She saw what she expected to see.

<u>Bad Idea #1</u>: When Rebecca felt chilly, sweaty, queasy or headachy, she thought she was sick. When she was on occasion short of breath because she was nervous or light-headed or because she had not eaten on a hot day, she thought she was sick. When she was out of sorts, she thought she was sick. Any ambiguity in her condition left room for her to conclude that she was sick. It seemed to her she was always either getting sick, sick, or slowly getting over being sick.

<u>Bad Idea #2</u>: Any hesitation on the part of a doctor to diagnose or treat was taken as a sign of ignorance or indolence. An inability of the doctor to explain what some other doctor was reputed to have said-perhaps in a recent magazine article- was taken as an indication that her doctor was not as knowledgeable as the other doctor. If her doctor was not perturbed, as she was, by that discrepancy, it was taken as a sign of complacency.

C. <u>Selective memory:</u> Rebecca, again like everyone else, tended to remember those events that fit with her view of the world or of herself (not necessarily a favorable view) and forget all the rest.

<u>Bad Idea #1</u>. Rebecca remembered all the times she had become ill. She forgot virtually all the vastly greater number of times she thought she was ill but was not, or about to become ill but did not. In fact, she remembered some of these times with the conviction that she had become ill despite the contrary recollection of all of her family. The well-known fallibility of eyewitness testimony is explained in part by similar psychological mechanisms.

<u>Bad Idea #2</u>: The times that doctors treated Rebecca with neglect and condescension (and there were such times) were etched indelibly in her memory. The usual patience and skill that characterized most of her encounters with physicians were mostly forgotten. It was not simply that they went unnoticed because they were what one would ordinarily expect from a doctor: it was because they were <u>not</u> what Rebecca expected.

D. <u>Group mythology:</u> There are commonly held beliefs that seem to confirm any point of view to someone already inclined to that view. Common prejudice is an example.

<u>Bad Idea #1</u>: Most people would agree that some people are simply unlucky in matters of health. They have "poor resistance" to infectious diseases and are "very sensitive" to drugs, which, therefore, may make them sicker. Everyone Rebecca knew agreed with her that she was such a person.

<u>Bad Idea #2</u>: Who has not been misdiagnosed or mistreated by some doctor at some point in his or her life? Whenever Rebecca expressed her skepticism about doctors, people rushed forward to report personal incidents of their own or accounts in the press that taken collectively would make a person seem reckless simply to visit a physician let alone rely blindly on his judgment. Just exiting a doctor's office must be dangerous, judging from all the anecdotes I have heard of somebody dropping dead just then, right after being given a clean bill of health by their doctors.

E. <u>Overvalued subjective experience:</u> Certain accidents or traumatic experiences make such a great impression on people they cause them to exaggerate the likelihood of similar incidents happening again.

<u>Bad Idea #1&2:</u>The striking experience Rebecca had following her miscarriage could be summarized briefly:

1. She told her doctor that there was something seriously the matter with her.
2. He reassured her, patronized her, really, without bothering to examine her or take her complaints seriously.
3. A moment later her doctor was talking and acting as if she were in immediate danger of dying.

Could anyone, no matter how poised or comfortable with herself, come away from such an encounter without thinking, first of all, that doctors cannot be trusted and, secondly, that life-perhaps her life in particular-is likely to vanish suddenly without warning? Had she only witnessed a medical emergency of this sort occurring to a friend or a relative, it might have influenced her similarly.

Most important: these Bad Ideas constitute self-confirming prejudices. Someone who already has a Bad Idea tests out the world in such a way that the results seem to justify that belief. The inclination to behave inappropriately because of a previously formed Bad Idea is precisely what makes neurotic people neurotic.

<u>Bad Idea #1</u>: Because Rebecca thought she was especially likely to get sick, she avoided everyone who was sick and from whom she might catch something; and, still, every once in a while she became ill- proving just how very vulnerable she was even under the best circumstances. "Just my luck," she always said.

<u>Bad Idea #2</u>: Not trusting doctors, Rebecca was in the habit of going from one to the other, asking one to confirm the judgment of the other, then asking searching questions to check one doctor's explanation against the other's. Invariably she discovered some small discrepancy which had to be resolved with expensive tests and further consultations. Often she exhausted her doctors' patience. She concluded none of them really knew

what they were talking about.

It was in such ways that Rebecca's fears were sustained over time. Her worries were exclusively about her health; but in many other people health anxiety overlaps with phobias and with other fears. There is a common denominator to these emotional disorders, which is the reason why they tend to appear in varying degrees in the same people. Such people have learned an attitude of vigilance. Sometimes the cause is a single traumatic incident. In my experience, though, it is the constant exposure throughout childhood to parental warnings, so ordinary they may go unchallenged and sometimes even unremembered, that have the most long-lasting effect. Overt symptoms of anxiety may begin, however, only years later.

The course of health anxiety is somewhat unpredictable. It may come in the wake of a particular physical illness and disappear subsequently for long periods of time only to become apparent again in the context of another minor illness. Or it may dominate and ruin most days of someone's life over a period of many years. Until recently, it was felt to be resistant to psychological treatment, partly because health worriers may not see themselves as emotionally disturbed and refuse, therefore, to enter treatment. When the condition appears secondary to depression, as it often does, it may very well disappear with the successful treatment of the underlying depression.

Some clinicians feel that people are born with a genetic vulnerability to all of the anxiety disorders. It may be so. Anyone who has examined new-born babies will have noticed that some children are much more reactive than others. Within the first few years of life, there are already noticeable differences in sociability or sensitivity to change. Even at this early state, one might conclude that some children are more likely to be easily frightened than others. But, in my opinion, the specific fears that trouble adults are always learned, in subtle ways, perhaps, but in the same ways that other facets of personality develop. And they can be unlearned. People can be taught to experience the world and themselves, and their bodies, in ways that allow them to be realistic and to put aside, finally, morbid concerns.

The Anxiety & Phobia Center
White Plains Hospital Center

Chief Complaint _____

Tentative Diagnosis _____

HEALTH ANXIETY SCALE

	Yes	No
Do you feel that you are likely to get sick more frequently than others, or are likely to get sicker than others when you do get sick?		
Do you think a lot about the possibility of getting illnesses that run in your family?		
When you develop physical symptoms, do you immediately contemplate the most serious illness that could explain these symptoms?		
Do you often think how terrible it would be for you or your children if you were to die prematurely?		
Are you under the impression that it is very important to get to a doctor at the first sign of getting sick?		
Do you visit doctors much more frequently than you really need to in order to be reassured about your health?		
Do you avoid doctors because you are frightened about what they might discover?		
Do you leave the doctor's office sometimes unsure of what he said or meant because you were nervous when he spoke to you?		
Although you know medical opinions can never be certain, do you nevertheless ask your doctor questions such as "are you sure I don't have ... cancer ... or AIDS ... or high blood pressure, etc.?" Is it hard for the doctor to reassure you?		
Do you ask what the cause of a symptom is even when the doctor has told you that that symptom is inconsequential?		

Do you ask your doctor to do medical tests in order "to be sure" even if the doctor is not otherwise inclined to order such tests?		
Do you worry for days ahead of time about routine tests such as a mammogram?		
Do you worry when a laboratory test result falls outside the normal range?		
Do you hesitate to take prescribed medicines because of concern about side effects?		
Are you more sensitive to medication than other people?		
Are you more inclined to take "natural" substances, such as herbs, rather than prescribed medicines?		
Do you worry when you have trouble sleeping or if your bowels are irregular?		
Do you check parts of your body over and over again looking for an abnormality such as a lump?		
Do you often suffer palpitations?		
Do you ask other people, such as a spouse, whether you are looking a little better today or a little worse?		
Do you worry about germs or about catching someone else's illness?		
Do you worry about very unlikely diseases such as a brain aneurysm that tend to lurk silently and may suddenly kill you?		
Are you preoccupied much of the time with thoughts of becoming ill or dying to the point, sometimes, where family members feel obligated to reassure you?		
Do you feel your health worries are foolish?		

Chapter Two: What Underlies Health Anxiety?

The way people respond to a situation is colored and often determined by their prior beliefs, which are in turn influenced by the thoughts and feelings of the people around them. For example, someone on a boat surrounded by people who are throwing up is likely herself to become sea sick. Similarly, discovering that one has eaten an unconventional food, (say, a grub) is enough to make that person feel nauseated suddenly. The "sick building syndrome," in which people who work inside a closed building fall ill, is due in part to the contagion of an idea. Being in a room where the windows will not open suggests that there is no ventilation; and even when the change of air through the ventilation system is greater than it would be with open windows, epidemics of sore throat, cough, and a general debilitation can spread throughout the building. A similar, well-publicized commotion took place not long ago when a group of toll-takers <u>on an open highway</u> got sick simultaneously from an unknown and, it turned out, nonexistent pollutant. Even yawning is contagious. People believe that they can be affected by invisible toxins or poisons in the air; and, of course, such things can and do happen.

But the fact that some people feel subjectively certain that they are allergic, or hyperreactive somehow does not make it so. There are people who believe they are so allergic to unknown chemicals in the air, or poisons in newsprint, that they have moved to the desert where they live in houses sheathed in plastic. Many parents are utterly convinced that their children become hyperactive after eating food additives, or even sugar, when investigations under double-blind conditions have proven conclusively that in fact no such effect exists. They report the same behavior whether their children are ingesting these substances or a placebo. There are many examples of mass hallucinations; hundreds of people have seen the face of Jesus in a cloud or on a tree trunk, and thousands have seen flying saucers, not to mention all those who have memories of being taken aboard those saucers forcibly by aliens from other planets! There has recently been described a false memory syndrome in which influential persons such as ministers or psychotherapists have elicited memories in others of events such as sexual abuse that in many cases <u>could not</u> have happened.

The truth is we remember what we are encouraged to remember, perceive what we expect to perceive, and feel the way we expect to feel. This commonplace observation is easy for us to accept about others, but very difficult to accept about ourselves. When we remember something clearly, when we feel something definitely, we stubbornly resist the need to stand outside ourselves and try to understand ourselves realistically by more objective means. When our lives are impaired by these beliefs, though, we must try. Probably in some ultimate sense, this task is impossible; but to some extent we can learn anew. First, it is helpful to be explicit about biases.

Health worriers share a number of dysfunctional ideas about the world. These Bad Ideas may not be conscious, but they are implicit in their behavior. Below is an attempt to make them explicit. Some of these ideas are inculcated during and throughout childhood, and so are hard to dispel. Others may not be so intractable. They may not be so much an expression of character as simply an outgrowth of being misinformed, sort of like thinking Milwaukee is in the southern hemisphere.

Bad Ideas of Health Worriers
1. <u>About physical illness</u>

Molly, who was 23 years old, had visited a doctor's office on five occasions in the previous five months, each time with a different complaint. She was playing tennis in May and wrenched her back. The thought occurred to her that she may have ruptured a spinal disk. She had a friend drive her immediately to the doctor. The pain resolved after a few days of bed rest and aspirin. In June she had a cold and a "stuffy" feeling in one ear. She returned from vacation early to visit the doctor and determine whether she had an ear infection, which she did not. She asked for antibiotics for her cold but was refused medication as unnecessary. Her cold subsided a few days later without additional treatment. In July her period came late. The thought occurred to her that she might have an ovarian tumor like her sister-in-law. After two days of waiting anxiously, she returned to the doctor, who once again prescribed no treatment. She menstruated two days later. A hot August caused her to feel light-headed, especially when she stood up suddenly. She immediately went to the doctor to rule out a brain tumor. He chose only to reassure her, but she continued to worry until September brought cooler temperatures, and she felt better. Late in September, however, while under the stress of giving a piano recital, she had an episode of abdominal cramps, which brought her quickly to the doctor's office with thoughts of colon cancer. Once again, her symptoms resolved quickly without medication.

Judging from Molly's actions, which are typical of health worriers, we might conclude that Molly believes:

A. That any illness, perhaps most of them, is potentially serious.
B. That the treatment of such an illness should be undertaken urgently to avoid dire consequences.
C. That most illnesses do not go away untreated
D. That the ordinary physical symptoms of anxiety, including stomach distress, light-headedness and vague physical pains, are more likely in her case to be caused by a serious illness.

The truth is: the great majority of illnesses cause no serious problems. They go away in a relatively short period of time without treatment. A few others linger but are not life-threatening. The reasons for visiting a doctor when acutely ill are two: first, to get palliative treatment in order to feel more comfortable while waiting for the condition to go away or, if it is chronic, to subside to its usual level, and, secondly, to rule out those few serious illnesses which do require prompt treatment. Even among those diseases which are serious, there are very few, putting aside injuries, that require treatment so urgently that it makes sense to go to a hospital emergency room in the middle of the night. Of course, a heart attack is one such condition. Is it helpful to know that most conditions are harmless when you know also that the one you think you may actually have may kill you? I hope so. Knowing the odds tends to reassure, although less than it should. Most health worriers can be told reliably that the odds against their having a heart attack are very long. It should be understood, at least, that the symptoms of a heart attack or any other serious disease bear little relationship to those symptoms of anxiety that are described above.

2. Bad Ideas about diet and sleep and the way the body functions in general.

Harold's parents had always been uneasy about his health, perhaps because he had been born prematurely. They made sure when he was growing up to guard him against extremes of temperature such as cold drafts. They made sure he ate properly and drank enough fluids. They emphasized the importance of being the right weight; and at various times they told him he was too fat and then, just a little later, too skinny. He continued to think about these things when he was an adult. He watched his weight, which was always too high, scrupulously. He limited his intake of spices. He was so worried about getting a good night's sleep, he found it difficult to fall asleep; and he became concerned if he had this problem three or four nights in a row. Similarly, he monitored the size and shape of his stool and worried about colon cancer if he did not move his bowels every day. He was incredulous when told that some people moved their bowels only once a week. He worried when his urine seemed too concentrated. He would not exercise if it was too hot or too cold. He would not swim after eating or taking a nap. He stayed out of the sun. He gargled frequently and brushed his tongue every day with a toothbrush. Any deviation from the "normal" pattern of bodily function started him worrying about the possibility of getting sick. For similar reasons he stayed away from sick people. Explicitly, he thought:

1. If you do not sleep eight hours every night, you will get sick.
2. If you do not eat three proper meals each day, you will get sick.
3. If you do not get enough rest, each and every day, you will get sick.
4. If you expose yourself in an intemperate manner to the elements, you will get sick.
5. If you visit somebody who is sick, you will get sick.

To sum up: he believed that physical health is precarious; and if you are not careful, you will get sick. Because there is a specific treatment program for insomnia these Bad Ideas are discussed again in Chapter 10.

The truth is: we have evolved as a species equipped to deal with the commonplace experiences of fasting, exposure to extremes of weather, and going without sleep. None of these predispose to serious physical illness. The reasons why doctors, who should know about such things, do not avoid sick people is that most illnesses, even contagious diseases, are not easy to catch. Of course, contagious diseases are communicated by more or less close contact with sick people, but the odds of catching most of these are not appreciably higher sitting in a sick room than they are in general. Of course, there are certain very serious illnesses, such as tuberculosis, which require special precautions, but these illnesses are few.

3. Bad Ideas about doctors

James was a 45-year-old man who had been ill for a period of a few weeks with a cough that seemed unresponsive to antibiotics and various cough medicines. He went to his own doctor a number of times, to an ear-nose-throat specialist, and to an expert on infectious diseases. Different diagnostic procedures had been performed, including throat cultures and chest x-rays and, at James' request, sinus x-rays and a CAT scan of the lungs. All had proven negative. Nevertheless, James was not comfortable with the unanimous advice of his physicians at this point to wait a while to see if his sore throat would clear by itself.

James entered then into the practice of calling one or another of his physicians every day, sometimes more than once. He reported to them subtle changes in his cough. One day he coughed a little more upon awakening than during the rest of the day. His mucous, which he examined carefully, had a greenish cast. On hot days his cough got worse, unless it was a dry, hot day. The antihistamines he took on his own made the cough better some days, but worse on other days. If he tilted his head off the side of the bed, the cough got worse for a while. Taking a deep breath made him cough more; and he took a deep breath frequently to make sure.

When his doctors failed to return his calls promptly, he became angry. Sometimes he called them at their homes, which made them angry. When they seemed not to be interested in his latest bulletin, he complained about their indifference. When they had no further tests to suggest or treatment to recommend, he complained about their ignorance. He was particularly incensed when his doctors offered vaguely dissimilar reasons for his cough. "A mild allergic bronchitis." "Postnasal drip."

"I've had this damn cough for months", he told his wife. "By now they should have been able to figure out what was causing it and what to do about it." It was another six months before the cough disappeared.

James believed that:

1. If a patient comes to a doctor, the doctor, if he is competent, should at the very least be able to tell the patient why he is feeling sick.

2. The doctor should be able to prescribe a drug or some other treatment that will remove the physical symptom and, for that matter, usually cure the underlying disease.

3. The doctor needs to know the exact shape of the symptom-what time of day did it manifest itself, did it change with eating, did it worsen with stress-to come to an expert judgment.

4. The doctor should be interested in the changing subtleties of the patient's complaints.

5. Considering the patient's distress, the doctor should be available to talk to him most of the time and should find something to say that will comfort and reassure.

6. Most doctors, however, are not interested, not caring, and not thorough. They are not sympathetic, and their judgment cannot be trusted.

7. Doctors are vague, and they contradict each other because they do not know, really, what they are talking about.

The ambivalent and troubled relationship of health worriers with their doctors is so central to their emotional problems that it is part of the definition of the illness; and I discuss this subject in detail in Chapter 5. It should be said here, though, that the health worrier's expectations from his or her doctor are unrealistic.

The truth is: Doctors are not able to explain every symptom that a patient has. Most illnesses disappear undiagnosed and perhaps undiagnosable. Neither are they as knowledgeable or, on the other hand, as incompetent as doctors may at various times seem. Most doctors are responsive to their patients and caring, but neither can it be said that they are as concerned about their patients' health to the extent that their patients are. As this book points out on every other page, often the patients worry more than they should.

4. Bad Ideas about drugs: Drugs have such central importance, they are discussed again in Chapter 10.

By the time Geraldine reached middle age, she had been in treatment with a number of psychiatrists and had seen very many other doctors for a variety of physical symptoms. On the most recent occasion she was found to be clinically depressed and, in the opinion of the psychiatrist she had consulted, needed to be on medication. So informed, Geraldine took out a list of medicines she had been on in the past, all with bad results. She thought that sometimes she had come close to dying.

There were eight anti-depressants listed, including all the newer serotonergic agents that are most commonly prescribed. They all caused jumpiness, sleeplessness, and "weird feelings," and were stopped, usually on Geraldine's insistence, after only a few days. A number of major tranquilizers had been prescribed for her in the past. These had more or less similar effects, except for one drug which made her feel better and then, when tried a second time, did not. A number of antibiotics caused rashes or stomach upset. Aspirin-like drugs caused cramps. It was her habit to start taking medicines in very small doses to get used to them, but usually even those sub-clinical doses caused untoward reactions of one sort or another. The only drug she got used to and then grew to depend on was Valium, a minor tranquilizer. She always carried some around "in case."

With these experiences in mind, Geraldine summed up her ambivalent attitude to drugs as follows:
"Believe me, I wish there was a drug I could take to make everything go away; but I can't. The drugs make it worse. I always take a half or a quarter of what I'm supposed to, and still my body is too sensitive. I know I have some kind of chemical imbalance that makes me react the wrong way, but nobody can find the right drug. Besides, drugs are dangerous."

Explicitly, she thought:
1. Drugs are very potent. Consequently:
  A. Any time you take a new drug, you are likely to get an allergic

reaction, like anaphylactic shock, which causes your bronchials to close up so that you choke to death in a few minutes. Otherwise you can get giant hives, some of which can land on your larynx, causing you to choke to death in a few minutes. There are other drug reactions in which the bone marrow is suppressed, causing death over a period of a few days or weeks. There are all kinds of other drug reactions possible in which death is only an unlikely, but disconcerting, possibility.

Therefore:

I. Do not take drugs unless you absolutely have to. Read the drug inserts first so you know what sort of drug reactions to expect.

II. If you do take drugs, you have to monitor your body especially carefully, looking in particular for headaches, dizziness and queasiness. It is good to take the least amount of drugs possible since doctors tend to prescribe too much.

B. Since there are so many potent drugs, there must be a drug to drive away my particular symptoms and relieve my particular condition; and if my doctor were clever and caring, he would give it to me.

C. Even if a drug, often a tranquilizer, does not seem to be helping, even if the doctor thinks it should be stopped, you had better keep taking it, or else. At least you should carry it around for a few years, just in case.

The truth is: It is not sensible to have an attitude about drugs per se, including the commonsense notion that you should not take drugs unless you really need them. After all, it is reasonable for most people most of the time to take aspirin for a headache even if the headache would have gone away eventually anyway. Drugs are tools, like a fork or an electric stove. They have to be judged each time, each one, on their merits. The purposes of drugs vary in importance. Some are trivial; but sometimes drugs are life-saving. They vary in their effectiveness at achieving their goal. Their side-effects vary. Luckily, dangerous allergic reactions are rare. The disadvantages of

42

taking drugs, which include not only side-effects, but, in some cases, an emotional dependence, must be measured each time against their advantages. No one who is competent should be forced to take medication against his or her wishes, however ill-judged that decision might be. On the other hand, that decision should not be made by the patient reading the insert that comes in the drug package. Mentioned on those pages (in really small writing) is every side-effect that has ever been reported with the use of the drug; but crucial information - namely, the frequency of those side-effects - is usually left out. Physicians make their recommendations after weighing all these considerations in the context of a particular patient with a particular illness and who may be on other drugs that can affect the metabolism of these drugs, and vice versa. As more drugs come into use, these decisions are becoming more difficult.

Although more drugs appear every year, there is not yet a drug for every symptom and every purpose. Patients should not feel entitled to a medication for every complaint. It should go without saying that medicines should be taken in the dosage prescribed. Either more or less may be dangerous. Asthmatics, for instance, have been reported recently to be endangering their lives by taking too little of one kind of medication and too much of another.

Since many health worriers are disgruntled by the lack of effectiveness of conventional treatment, they may - like terminal cancer patients - be inclined to try unproved and unscientific treatments, ranging from chiropractic to "blood cleansing." These go under the rubric sometimes of "holistic medicine," by which these adherents mean to suggest that they treat all of the patient rather than merely his disease. Some recommend homeopathic medicine, which is out and out magic, medicine diluted often to such an extent that none of it is left! Holistic practitioners also emphasize nutrition, which is indeed important, but only rarely important in the treatment of acute illnesses other than nutritional states. Nevertheless, it is not unusual for someone to convince himself or herself that such a treatment may be effective.

A 27 year old man named Seymour was a body-builder and, to use his characterization, a "health nut." He was very careful about what he put in his body, he said. In fact, he ate hardly any food. His diet consisted of protein additives and high-caloric drinks. He also took handfuls of vitamin pills 3 or 4 times a day. As a result, he never got colds, he informed me - although he was sniffling and sneezing throughout our conversation! The fact is, he was relatively healthy, although probably no more so than most people his age.

Ephraim was not so lucky. When he was 24, a doctor told him to take a multivitamin four times a day. He did so for the next 40 years, at which time he presented on a neurology service with convulsions. He was suffering from vitamin D poisoning, which had caused calcium to precipitate out in his kidneys, skin and brain.

Even acupuncture, which is widely accepted, has not yet really proven its effectiveness – even for the treatment of pain, let alone the more exotic uses to which it is put, such as increasing sexual potency. Unconventional treatments may turn out to be useful, but most of them will not. They work, insofar as they do work, because of the placebo effect. When the placebo effect wears off, as it does usually in a matter of days or weeks, the health worrier is left more distraught and more cynical than before.

5. <u>Bad Ideas about physical examinations and laboratory tests</u>.

Alberta was a very outspoken and self-assured young woman, except when it came to her health. Even there, she had developed some fixed ideas about what constituted proper medical care; and that was what she demanded. For example, one time when she had experienced abdominal cramps off and on for a couple of days, she visited her doctor and was annoyed when the physician was unable immediately to arrive at a definitive diagnosis. She was further annoyed that her examination did not include looking into her ears and testing her deep tendon reflexes. She requested a "total body scan," just in case something obscure was going wrong somewhere. She had in mind some other blood tests that had not occurred to her doctor, such as a 5-hour glucose tolerance test. When the doctor pointed out that this test would not bear on her stomach complaints, she threatened to go elsewhere. As was usually the case with Alberta, her doctor agreed finally to satisfy her wishes in order to placate her and possibly reassure her. When the test came back just slightly out of the usual range, she demanded to know why. When he could not tell her, she left his office peremptorily and his practice. She went from one doctor to the next, sometimes because she was asked to leave.

Explicitly, Alberta thought that if an illness is present:

A. A really complete physical examination should pick up signs of it, especially if that examination is conducted at a time when symptoms are present. Symptoms, although subjective, should be apparent somehow on examination.

B. A really good examination should include all of the body, no matter what complaint the patient has. Similarly, laboratory tests should test for everything.

C. Any deviation from the usual in bodily function or appearance is obviously abnormal and should be pursued by the doctor and explained. Similarly, any laboratory results that are reported back as being outside normal limits are by definition abnormal. It is sensible to think that these results may be related to the patient's complaints, whatever they are.

D. If there is a laboratory investigation or procedure that could conceivably explain the patient's symptoms, it should be done as soon as possible and, possibly, repeated, just to be sure.

E. A CAT scan or an MRI is a good test to do, no matter what.

The truth is: that medical diagnosis is based more on the patient's account of his or her symptoms than on the results of physical examination, which, like any other investigation, is more likely to be successful when one knows ahead of time what to look for. See Chapter 5. Often, when someone is sick, there are no objective signs apparent. Symptoms are always subjective and may very well not have a physical corollary. <u>A negative physical examination does not mean to the doctor that a physical symptom is not real or is in some way imaginary.</u>

Similarly, with the exception of a few routine screening tests, laboratory tests should be performed only with the intention of looking for a particular result in order to rule out particular diseases. These are diseases or disease processes that are suggested by the patient's complaints. There are more and more tests available all the time, literally thousands. They are time-consuming and expensive and serve inevitably to focus the health worrier's attention increasingly on his or her physical complaints. This result is directly opposite to the goals of treatment for this emotional disorder. The mere act of investigating the patient's health is counter-therapeutic and should be undertaken only for specific goals and <u>not</u> "just to be sure," especially since certainty in matters of health can never be obtained. Also, some laboratory procedures are risky. Yet, doctors are often convinced by stubborn patients to order tests that carry a measurable morbidity. A number of patients have undergone coronary angiography, a complicated, expensive and invasive test for coronary artery disease, when the patient had no symptoms to suggest coronary artery disease!

The truth is, also, that variations from the usual on physical examination, or in laboratory tests, may not have any relevance to the patient's condition. There are, for example, functional murmurs of the heart that have no clinical significance. All laboratory tests and diagnostic procedures have less than perfect sensitivity and specificity. See Chapter 6. For that reason alone, and for others, tests have meaning only in the context of a particular patient.

The CAT scan (computerized axial tomography) and the M.R.I. (magnetic resonance imaging) are marvelous tests, although expensive, which allow doctors to see inside the body in arbitrarily defined cross-sections. There are other tests using sound echoes that do something similar. Certain tests are better at finding particular structural abnormalities than others; and one may be used in preference to others depending on what kind of information is being sought. No test, no matter how good, is best in every situation. A test may be more informative performed at one point in a patient's illness rather than another. And so the decision to order a test at one time or another must be medically informed. Often it is necessary to wait. <u>Often waiting to see what happens to the patient's symptoms is the best test of all</u>. However, doctors, subject to pressure like anyone else, tend to order tests prematurely on anxious patients who wish to make certain that they are not seriously ill. The impossible, implacable search for certainty is the hallmark of obsessive-compulsive disorder, of which health anxiety is one form. Continual testing worsens the condition and often, as a matter of fact, supplies no new information.

<u>Bad Ideas about death and dying</u>. See Chapter 14.

It has often been said that the fear of death is basic and underlies all other fears. But anyone who listens closely to health worriers will realize that other fears, still more basic, drive their concerns about becoming ill and most of all becoming ill with a fatal illness. Each person mentioned below said he or she was afraid of developing a fatal illness. At first glance it appeared they were all afraid of the same thing; but they were not.

A young man was afraid of dying prematurely from a heart attack because he thought his children would have no one (except their mother) to take care of them.

A young mother who had panic attacks was afraid of fainting (or dying) suddenly and having her small children wander off into danger.

A middle-aged woman whose parents had been divorced

when she was a child was afraid of developing a deadly disease because she thought her family could not be relied on to take care of her in the end.

An elderly bachelor was afraid of being overcome by a stroke which would leave him lying helpless on the floor unable to reach a telephone.

Others are afraid of wasting away and becoming ugly or helpless. Still others are afraid of the pain of terminal cancer. Some are afraid of losing their minds or simply of being unable to control their bodily functions, and losing their dignity. Not a few are afraid of their doctors. Some are afraid of being buried alive. But, if asked, all said they were afraid of dying.

Explicitly, a health worrier may think that: The process of dying is usually painful and sometimes intolerably painful. Hospitals are terrible, impersonal places where dying patients are ignored, and tormented with needles the rest of the time. Each day brings more bad news. Friends and family visit less and less frequently because they too feel awful. Doctors are arbitrary and the dying person is helpless to resist them. Inherent in dying is the loss of autonomy and self-respect and, finally, the loss of hope. The fatal illness, which may have already begun, will worsen slowly along with the person's terror until, in a final anguish, all alone, the person dies.

<u>The truth is:</u> it is hard to put a nice face on death, and I will not try. It is, surely, a final ending, an end to struggle and planning and worry, and everything with which we busy our lives - but not really to everything in our lives. Children live on. Sometimes the work we have done - or other things that mattered to us - continues on. This makes a difference psychologically. Some people die content. The deaths different people suffer are as different as the lives they have lived; but it is a fact that most people die, perhaps tired, and even sometimes regretful, even bitter, but rarely afraid. With modern medicines there is no reason for anyone to die in extreme pain; and

most people do not. They still die uncomfortable deaths, often with needles and tubes and a pointless agitation on many hospital wards; but it need not be so. The particular scenarios of death that health worriers imagine are important in understanding them as people, but they are not realistic. Doctors and nurses find it hard dealing with dying patients, but they are not indifferent to their patients' needs; and they are still subject to their patients' wishes. A dying person is still in control of his or her life. The small remainder of life can be lived with dignity and self-respect. Anyone who has friends and family will not die alone. It is those fears that underlie the fear of death: the fear of being alone and the fear of being helpless. How could it be otherwise? Death is an abstraction. Only a symbol. No one has experienced death. Its terror lies in its ability to call up images of a final and utter helplessness and loneliness. Those who feel sure that the people to whom they feel close will respond to them, will not fear death. One can learn not to be afraid of death as one can learn not to be afraid of the act of dying. Or of being sick enough to die.

The Bad Ideas that underlie health anxiety are taken up again in more detail in later chapters.

Chapter Three: The Worry Wheel

How do Bad Ideas crystallize at a particular time in someone's life into a full-blown health anxiety? And what sustains this disorder over time? What allows health worriers to become preoccupied with the possibility of being seriously ill when they are told repeatedly by experts that they are not seriously ill, and, often enough, told they are not ill at all?

As described in previous chapters, some people are brought up in subtle ways to be cautious in general and to worry about their health in particular. But such a point of view about themselves and about the world is merely an inclination to distort everything slightly in a particular direction, like looking though sunglasses all day long or like being a liberal or a conservative. No particular distress is involved, and health worriers, not yet actively worrying, have no reason to think there is anything the matter with them. They would have no trouble defending the Bad Ideas described in the last chapter. Those ideas seem reasonable to them. But at some particular time, often with little provocation, a circular process is set in motion which makes the worrier more and more distraught until he or she is chronically ill with what seems to the affected person, and to everyone close to that person, to be a significant emotional disorder.

Gavin claimed that he had never worried about his health until his older sister was diagnosed with psoriasis. He was surprised to learn that psoriasis can cause a number of different problems, including arthritis. He, himself, had been feeling vague joint pains, particularly in his knees after playing tennis. It made sense to him to check his skin for signs of psoriasis. Sure enough, he found some scaly patches around his nose and the back of his ears. He made an appointment the following week to see a dermatologist, but, in the meantime, found himself checking the back of his ears (with mirrors and with difficulty) frequently. Along the way, he noticed a mole on his back, which he began to worry about. He thought of the possibility of a malignant melanoma. A still more careful search revealed another flat, darkened mole on the sole of one foot, along with many other smaller moles that he had not noticed previously. At this time he happened to read that certain abdominal cancers can cause skin lesions; and, for that matter, certain skin cancers could spread and cause headaches and stomach aches. Recently, he had been having both headaches and stomach aches. He made a long overdue appointment to see his internist.

The dermatologist told Gavin that he had a seborrheic dermatitis on his face and behind his ears. Not psoriasis. He called the moles on his back and foot "transitional epitheliomas," which, he said, were unimportant, but which he admitted, after being pressed by Gavin, had a very small malignant potential. He also admitted grudgingly that Gavin had more than his share of moles in general and probably should be examined at intervals of six months or a year. Gavin was disturbed by the possibility of some of these moles becoming melanomas; and so the two that had troubled him particularly - on his back and foot - were removed, reluctantly, by the dermatologist.

The internist Gavin saw was similarly unimpressed by the severity of his other physical complaints; but the doctor recognized that, for whatever reason, Gavin was becoming increasingly upset. One reason, Gavin acknowledged, had nothing directly to do with his own health. He had recently taken an interest in the health of his neighbors and discovered there was what seemed to him an unusually large number of cancers in his immediate neighborhood. He had become concerned about the effects of pollution from an industrial plant in the next county. The doctor ordered a series of tests, which turned out negative.

It is difficult to summarize in a few paragraphs Gavin's complicated interaction with various doctors and hospitals over the next six months. Although every physician he saw was of the opinion he had nothing seriously the matter with him, he still underwent multiple x-ray studies, endoscopy of different sorts, one more skin biopsy, and many different blood studies. He was discovered to have a high blood bilirubin and a few red cells in his urine, both of which were regarded finally as not reflecting any medical disease, but only after provoking cystoscopy and other confirmatory blood studies. Gavin was left, finally, increasingly anxious about his health and with a growing number of physical symptoms, including worsening headaches, stomachaches and fatigue.

He was finally judged to be depressed.

We may call the process by which Gavin got more and more upset the Worry Wheel. See illustration 1, on facing page.

To begin with, there exists in an affected person a predilection to worry about health, although these concerns may be relatively mild and not always apparent in retrospect. Nor is it always the case that health worriers remember their parents as being the frightened people and inclined to frighten others that I have described here. Perhaps they are right. Other people besides parents can influence children when they are growing up. Sometimes there is a singular incident in these children's lives that made the sort of impression that is usually made most readily by parents repeatedly expressing their own fears. The child becoming seriously ill or the death of a close relative might be such a circumstance. Still, most of the time health worriers remember only that their parents also worried about health.

The trigger that sets the worry wheel in motion may be a sudden illness or the death of a relative or a friend. Sometimes it is an illness of the patient when that illness is unusual in some respect or hangs on for an unusually long period of time. Sometimes the mere coincidence of a famous person of the same age dying will start the process as will the patient reaching the age that one of his or her parents died. The onset of a depression, which can occur at any age with very little of an obvious precipitant, can cause physical symptoms, especially those associated with agitation and excitement, and

THE WORRY WHEEL

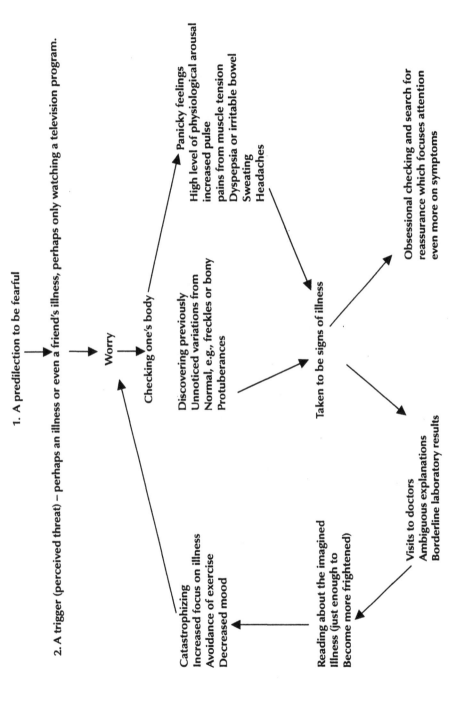

1. A predilection to be fearful

2. A trigger (perceived threat) – perhaps an illness or even a friend's illness, perhaps only watching a television program.

Worry

Checking one's body

Discovering previously
Unnoticed variations from
Normal, e.g., freckles or bony
Protuberances

Panicky feelings
High level of physiological arousal
increased pulse
pains from muscle tension
Dyspepsia or irritable bowel
Sweating
Headaches

Taken to be signs of illness

Obsessional checking and search for
reassurance which focuses attention
even more on symptoms

Visits to doctors
Ambiguous explanations
Borderline laboratory results

Reading about the imagined
Illness (just enough to
Become more frightened)

Catastrophizing
Increased focus on illness
Avoidance of exercise
Decreased mood

suggest to the affected person that he or she is physically ill. And so, the health worrier begins unequivocally to worry.

Somebody worried about losing his shirt in the stock market might find himself checking the market action repeatedly during the course of the day. Someone worried about a ballet performance she is going to give or an examination she is scheduled to take might very well run through her steps or check her classroom notes repeatedly. This sort of checking behavior seems understandable to us, and often serves the purpose of making a desired result more likely. Rehearsal is likely to improve performance; studying more and more is likely to result in a better grade. But the checking that a health worrier does is more like someone who is afraid his automobile battery had gone dead and tests it by starting the car, and starting it again and again until the battery is dead. A number of cases have been reported in the medical literature of people who have examined parts of their bodies so strenuously that these structures have become inflamed and had to be removed! These body parts include in one case a parotid gland and in another a testicle.

Helen was one of a great number of women who worry about breast cancer to an extent way out of proportion to the risk it represents. However, she seemed more concerned about the cosmetic effect of a mastectomy than a possible threat to her life. In any case, she examined her breasts almost continually. She had a tendency to fibrocystic disease, which was, according to her doctor, aggravated by her prodding and probing. As a consequence, her breast tissue had become so thickened, it was no longer possible to do a proper breast examination without coming across a number of lumps.

Health worriers check:
1. Their pulse and blood pressure. Since the pulse varies with excitement and nervousness, no useful information is obtained, even in the unlikely event that the heart rate might otherwise be

relevant to the patient's complaints. Besides, the heart rate varies very widely within a normal range. The mere fact of taking one's pulse will raise it. So much is true also about blood pressure, which is less readily checked by a lay person, although worriers have purchased sphygomanometers for this purpose. Repeated blood pressure readings are not useful except in those circumstances where the patient is hypertensive and is told by the doctor to perform these examinations at home. In any case, the symptoms a health worrier has are not likely to be caused by hypertension which is largely an asymptomatic disease throughout most of its course.

2. Their breathing. Breathing is a self-regulating, largely unconscious process; and it, too, varies with emotional distress and also with activity level, sexual arousal and a half-dozen other influences. Paying attention to one's breathing changes breathing, usually by accelerating it. The syndrome of hyperventilation, in which people overbreathe, is caused by the anxious person having a sense of not being able to catch his or her breath. As a consequence, excess carbon dioxide is exhaled, changing the acid-base balance of the blood, causing calcium to ionize, which produce a tetany-like state with tingling of fingers and lips and a strange, muscular cramping of the hands - all of which serve, as one might expect, to considerably worsen the anxious person's distress. A common treatment for hyperventilation is to offer the patient a paper bag to breath into, thereby preventing the excessive loss of carbon dioxide. Dramatic though this syndrome is, it is self-limiting and reversible, so I do not recommend this treatment, which serves to focus attention still more on breathing, and makes the patient feel ridiculous in the bargain.

3. Their sense of balance. Walking with perfect balance is made impossible by concentrating on balance, just as attempting to sign one's name especially clearly produces a signature different from the usual "normal" one.

4. Their ability to see clearly. Since we all have two eyes, and they do not see equally well, it is easy comparing one against the other to imagine a deterioration of function. Many people have "floaters," little spots that seem to move to and fro in the field of vision. These usually have no significance but are troubling to the health worrier.

5. Their ability to think or remember. Everyone complains of a memory not as good as it used to be, maybe because there is more to remember as time goes on. In any case, memory can be expected to suffer in any situation where a person is distracted by pain or by any strong feeling at all, such as depression or grief, or romantic love, for that matter. Worsening memory does not imply organic brain disease. At a time of my life when I could have been described reasonably as young middle-aged, I had a dream in which I could not remember the name of Alzheimer's disease. I woke up in the middle of the night and was disconcerted to find that I still could not remember the name. I was sufficiently troubled to start searching through the index of a neurology textbook-alphabetically, luckily. I did not grow more forgetful in later years.

6. Their digestion. Some people spend considerable time examining their urine, their stool or their menstrual flow for irregularities of color or shape. All three are influenced by emotional distress and, of course, all three vary for all sorts of trivial reasons. Dyspepsia and cramping are common and commonly associated with anxiety. Dyspepsia, more recently called GERD (gastroesophageal reflux disorder), but more usually called heartburn, is made worse by the air swallowing that accompanies anxiety. So is cramping. Cramps and gas pains are often associated with loose stools and/or constipation, and are usually called irritable bowel syndrome.

7. Their skin. For lumps, moles and discolorations.

8. Their sexual functioning. The ability to function sexually is

impaired by testing the ability to function sexually too frequently over too brief a period of time. Men more so than women. More directly, worrying about whether one will be able to get an erection in the next 5 minutes is not likely to encourage a favorable result.

9. Finally, whatever pain they may have been experiencing recently for changes in quality. If the health worrier checks for tenderness in the temporal-mandibular joint often enough, the joint tends to become inflamed. Pain changes, anyway, from day to day for unimportant reasons, or, at least, reasons that are less important than those the health worrier can imagine.

Many of the symptoms described above come in the wake of anxiety or by testing bodily functions in such a way as to disturb them. See Chapter 12 for a discussion of those physical symptoms produced solely from the effects of stress. But, it is true, also, that once the worry wheel is set in motion, the health worrier notices bodily defects that were always present but unnoticed until this time.

It was inevitable that I would suffer a bad case of "medical student's disease" when that time came. Once I thought I had an acute intestinal obstruction. It turned out to be gas. Later on I noticed a bony protuberance on the lateral aspect of my leg just below the knee. It occurred to me with a pang that bony cancers occur most commonly there, at the ends of the long bones. I was comforted at once, though, taking note that I had a similar bump on the other leg. Even I could not entertain the fiction that I had simultaneously developed matching sarcomas in two different places. I was bow-legged. The bumps had always been there, unnoticed, and are there still.

Everyone has bony protuberances, or a pattern of freckles or spots, that are simply a variation of normal; but should they be discovered near an area of recent concern, they are likely to be regarded by the health worrier as one more sign of a significant problem.

In such ways, checking one's body, perhaps with the vague wish to reassure oneself, serves paradoxically to frighten. No one functions with the regularity of a clock. The ordinary and common-place disturbances described above are taken to be signs of illness by the health worrier, who examines himself or herself with the hope of finding a perfect, unblemished symmetry and regularity of function, and always finds something else. And, if, in fact, the health worrier does have a minor illness, there are always more specific symptoms to monitor: fever, or cough, perhaps, along with pain.

Not so bad cases (N.S.B.)

Charlie, who had no prior history of serious physical illness, or concern about physical illness, came home from a vacation one summer tired and with a stomach condition diagnosed as a gastroenteritis. His stomach problem cleared in time, but his excessive fatigue remained. He also complained about a mild dizzyness. During the next few months, he went to a number of doctors, who made a number of different diagnoses, including an inner ear disorder. As the months wore on, and he experienced no improvement, he began to worry that he had a serious illness the doctors were missing. Finally, he took a new job, which distracted him, and his symptoms and his concern about them faded without treatment.

Suzanne had no health worries until she attempted to become pregnant at the age of 34. When she did not readily conceive, she went to a doctor who put her through a battery of tests. He discovered a number of "genetic abnormalities," none of which caused her any discomfort or contributed to her difficulty becoming pregnant. They included an IGA deficiency (a common immunological defect), a minor thalassemia (causing small red blood cells), and a persistent high bilirubin, (Gilbert's Syndrome - of no clinical significance.) Along the way, a suspicious mole was discovered and removed. Suzanne developed an exaggerated concern about her body temperature and her health in general. And this did not go away until she gave birth a year later.

Ned was one of those people who felt they were always having to contend with stressful circumstances, in his case, particularly on the job. Because he was panicky from time to time, his physician put him on antidepressant medication. A few months later, a routine laboratory test showed that he had a somewhat low platelet count. Very low platelets can cause bleeding. Ned was troubled a little by this possibility, but so was his doctor, who immediately stopped the anti-depressants, which had been reported in the past very rarely to depress platelets. Repeated tests showed no increase in the platelet level. Ned began to notice now that he had palpitations when he was particularly distressed; and he began to have trouble catching his breath. He worried that he might have asthma, which ran in his family. All of these worries disappeared after he read about asthma and when it was discovered by going through his old medical records that he had been running a low platelet count for the previous 10 years without untoward consequences.

Going to the Doctor

Being sick, and feeling sicker, it is reasonable to visit the doctor. Or is it? Throughout much of history a sick person would have been well-advised to stay as far away from medical treatment as possible. Between the practice of bloodletting and the use of purgatives and such, treatment was likely to worsen any condition rather than improve it. But in the last century the practice of medicine has become rational, that is, founded on scientific principles; and drugs that truly work have become available along with other effective treatments. Nevertheless, experience shows that most illnesses disappear just as quickly without any treatment. For that reason someone who wakes up one day with pain in a joint, or diarrhea, or a sore throat, or any of a great many other commonplace symptoms is likely to wait a while before visiting a doctor, acting on the expectation that a few days later those symptoms will be gone. If someone starts with the assumption that he will get better, it is reasonable to wait a while before seeing a doctor. On the other hand, if one expects to be still sicker a few days later, it is appropriate to visit a doctor as soon as possible. In practice, everyone follows more complicated rules. If a symptom is new and unfamiliar, or if it is worrisome because it suggests a serious illness such as cancer or heart disease, or simply because the person is very uncomfortable, it becomes sensible to go promptly to a physician. If going to a doctor reassures a worried patient, that result alone is worth the time and money. Unfortunately, when someone troubled by health anxiety visits a doctor, he or she is likely to come away more worried. The reasons for this paradoxical and perverse result are described in the next chapter. For purposes of explaining the worry wheel, the bottom line is this:

Health worriers go to the doctor(s) and come away feeling more anxious because:

1. They feel the doctor(s) did not really understand their physical complaints.
2. The doctor(s)' explanations of those complaints are vague and uncertain.
3. The laboratory results that were reported back were ambiguous.
4. The doctor(s) ordered further tests, the result of which will not be known until next week.
5. The doctors disagreed among themselves, suggesting that none of them really knows what they are talking about.
6. The doctor(s) insisted on "waiting to see" rather than doing those tests right now that might turn out to be definitive.
7. No doctor will guarantee absolutely that a very serious disease is not lurking somewhere under the surface.

Health worriers wait, then, impatiently for their latest laboratory results and their next doctor's appointment, meanwhile checking their bodies for signs that their illness may be progressing. If they have, in fact, been ill, they may feel slightly better as their cough lessens or as their pain recedes. If their symptoms disappear entirely, they may feel much better, only, suddenly, to hear on the radio a report of someone who just died after having a coughing spell or having pain just like theirs. And their cough returns. And their pain returns. They may read articles on precisely their condition – or the condition they suspect they may have – and all of their symptoms return.

As the worry wheel turns again and again, sooner or later the health worrier becomes demoralized and resentful, and often frankly depressed. Sometimes he or she may have started off depressed. A major depression often begins with physical symptoms. There are very effective treatments for depression, both psychological and pharmacological, but they require that the health worrier be willing to see himself or herself as troubled emotionally. Usually, however, most health worriers are caught up exclusively with the likelihood of a physical disease. Becoming depressed-and, of course, feeling sick too-the health worrier retreats from physical exercise and may take to bed. There are real physical consequences to excessive rest. They are the reason why patients are ambulated as quickly as possible in a hospital setting after surgery. Even major surgery. The vascular system relaxes, causing labile blood pressure and dizziness, sometimes fainting. Walking may be unsteady because of muscular weakness and mild vestibular dysfunction. Anyone who spends considerable time in bed but not sleeping invariably develops a sleeping problem. Appetite disturbances, sometimes to the extent of causing weight loss, may also ensue. Soon a melange of physical and emotional symptoms lead one into the other so that nobody, not the patient, not even a presumably objective physician, can tell what is causing what. The most characteristic physical symptom of depression or any other emotional disorder, and of most physical disorders too, is fatigue.

The chronic fatigue syndrome - which may be caused by one or another obscure virus, but which is usually not - closely resembles this clinical picture. The diagnosis is made when someone relatively abruptly develops a profound lack of energy and a variety of vague physical symptoms. The well-recognized treatment is a combination of anti-depressant medications and an exercise program. The doctors who are best able to convince patients to participate in such a difficult and uncongenial therapy are those who profess a belief in the illness being physically caused rather than psychological. Patients want to be taken seriously. Unfortunately, most people see physical disorders as more real than those that are emotional in origin. In real life these distinctions break down, for the reasons described above.

The different turns along the worry wheel provide points of attack for the treatment of health anxiety. Various misconceptions drive the health worrier's concerns at these various points; and these must be dispelled as far as possible. Perhaps chief among these are the Bad Ideas the patient has about the nature of physical illness, about medical treatment itself, and about what can reasonably be expected from a doctor.

Chapter Four: Real Physical Illness

Ideas about health can be very hard to change. Some patients believe absolutely that they have certain illnesses despite there being no evidence to support those diagnoses. For example, many such patients think they have hypoglycemia. Hypoglycemia, low blood sugar, causes certain symptoms: fatigue, shakiness, changes in mood, disorientation, and others, all of which taken together may be confused by an inexperienced observer with symptoms of the much more common anxiety disorders, in particular, panic disorder. True hypoglycemia is unusual and sometimes the consequence of a serious condition such as an insulin-producing tumor. Reactive hypoglycemia is a much less distinct disorder. Supposedly, some people react to a sugary meal by a rise and then a greater fall in blood sugar than usual. Blood levels considered normal by most endocrinologists are regarded by others as abnormally low. Those inclined to make the diagnosis make it frequently. The diagnosis is said to be in error 95% of the time. Other illnesses diagnosed carelessly are mitral valve prolapse, fibromyalgia, chemical sensitivity, chronic fatigue syndrome and chronic lyme disease. Many of these patients feel they are desperately ill and ignored by the medical establishment. On the other hand, some physicians, if they become convinced that a patient has hypoglycemia will make that diagnosis even when the blood level is within normal limits, explaining their opinion in terms of <u>the rate that the blood sugar drops!</u> Consequently, many patients with a variety of non-specific symptoms carry this diagnosis - wholeheartedly. They become convinced that they have a "real" physical disorder rather than an emotional condition, which in their mind would be trivial and not worthy of anyone's attention.

One such patient, a woman suffering from panic disorder, insisted to me that her symptoms were due instead to hypoglycemia. She could "feel" her blood sugar dropping right after an attack. She had taken to carrying around a carrot as a way of aborting the attack.

The fact that she misunderstood her symptoms and found comfort in a remedy that would not have been helpful to her even if she had hypoglycemia distracted us from dealing with the true causes of her panic disorder and prevented us from beginning appropriate treatment. I thought to demonstrate to her once and for all that her blood sugar level was normal during her attacks. Repeatedly, over the course of a week, I had her blood drawn at just those times. When all nine laboratory results were spread before her, all normal, she looked up at me and said the laboratory must be in error! Actually, two laboratories!

Another woman was convinced she was anemic because people kept telling her she looked pale. She dismissed repeated blood tests that indicated otherwise.

A young fellow, one of many, believed he was suffering from heart disease because he had pain on the left side of his chest. Three cardiologists reassured him after he had taken a number of tests, all of which were unnecessary even in their eyes, that his heart was fine. They pointed out that heart pain is typically mid-line and not in the left chest as one might naively think; but he remained troubled and unconvinced.

Another woman complained of intractable pain and could not believe that all the examinations and tests she underwent showed no apparent cause of it. There are many such patients. They feel that if a doctor says he cannot find the source of their pain, he is really saying that he does not believe that they are in pain. Sometimes, rarely I hope, that is what the doctor means. However, most doctors understand that there are many undefined and undiagnosable causes of pain. It is just this fact that patients have trouble understanding. Their having pain, or other symptoms for that matter, does not mean doctors can find a reason for it. Believing otherwise, however, patients may develop strained relationships with their physicians, trying to squeeze from them explanations they do not have. Most common of all, more the rule than the exception, are those who feel they are suffering from some obscure illness which their doctors are too unskilled or too careless to diagnose.

Some health worriers are convinced utterly that they can feel their blood coursing through their bodies or feel various hot and cold discharges along their nerves. Such things are not possible, but the sensation is so real, their conviction assumes almost delusional proportions. Their view might be summed to the idea "I know my body and I know what my body is telling me." It is very hard to convince them that their body might be telling them only what they expect to hear.

Health worriers adhere stubbornly to their ideas about their health - or ill health; but they are not altogether unreasonable. There are certain things worth knowing, facts about illness and about the practice of medicine, that health worriers do not know for the most part, that are surprising to them, and that, when understood, help them to achieve a more accurate perspective on their health. That is, they worry less.

Most people have a somewhat mistaken view of what it means to be sick. They imagine that they are usually entirely well until a particular thing happens, after which they fall ill. Everything happens for a reason; and so they expect that prompt medical attention will make that reason evident. The doctor will do a complete physical examination, the more detailed the better, order appropriate laboratory tests, no matter what the expense, and will come up with an appropriate diagnosis. For each illness, there is an appropriate remedy, which the doctor will prescribe. Shortly, they will once again be entirely well.

In real life people are never entirely well. Out of view, the immune system is always combating some problem or other; and the various systems that operate to maintain homeostasis are never entirely in balance. Sometimes for no discernible reason things get worse and an illness becomes apparent for the first time. Health worriers who get sick for no particular reason, who go undiagnosed after seeing many doctors and undergoing many tests, and who do not recover promptly, feel that something has gone wrong. Either they have some mysterious and, potentially serious disorder, or their doctor is incompetent. They expect too much. In some sense, they expect too little, since they do not expect to recover by themselves in the natural way of things. In fact, most illnesses differ from the health worrier's concept of illness in a number of important respects. These are the facts:

The usual course of physical illness

Of course, physical illnesses differ from each other. Some start suddenly, others more insidiously. Some are genetic and present from birth and throughout life. Others are genetic but only appear later on. There are many such illnesses including familiar ones such as gout and migraine. Some conditions give no sign of being present at all until they kill suddenly. Brain aneurysms and some heart attacks may have this character. Certain cancers also. These are especially frightening to health worriers since no one can assure them on the basis of an ordinary physical examination that they definitely do not have these disorders. On the other hand, infectious diseases sometimes do follow the simple model described in the last section. Some people can point to a time when they got sick and to another time approximately when they got well. However, many other infections, such as malaria, come and then come again and again. Certain forms of hepatitis come and never go away. Sometimes it is possible to determine just those circumstances under which an infection was contracted – venereal diseases, for instance. More often not. The familiar routine in which health worriers try to figure out whether they caught a cold from Aunt Celia yesterday or from Uncle Harry the day before is a waste of time. For one thing, a cold can be transmitted by someone who does not yet have symptoms. For another, the incubation of viral disease varies so greatly it is impossible to tell whether the illness was contracted yesterday or last week. Some illnesses develop months or years after the time of infection or longer. AIDS may become apparent only many years later. Where and when exactly someone gets sick, or how, for that matter, is usually beside the point anyway. A doctor may want to know if a patient has been out of the country recently since different infections are endemic in the different parts of the world, but once the diagnosis has been made the treatment is the same. The desire of health worriers to know exactly how and why they got sick comes out of the notion that illness is something that can be figured out exactly, something that came from someplace apart from themselves and that can, if treated properly, be removed.

In contrast to some infectious diseases, most illnesses described in medical textbooks are chronic. They get noticed for the first time at a particular time, but usually they were in the process of developing long before. Among them are some that are troublesome, but not usually life-threatening. These include arthritis, diabetes, hypertension, ulcerative colitis and many others. Most of these conditions are treatable but not curable. Their symptoms subside to some extent with proper treatment. For those affected by one of them, and as everyone else grows older almost everyone is, the illness fades after a while from their awareness. People instead concern themselves with the everyday matters that preoccupy them in general: family relationships, problems on the job, routine pleasures, and on. As more time passes, other illnesses develop, everything from cataracts to gum disease; and these too become unimportant although vexing from time to time. What seems unbelievable to health worriers is that the more serious, potentially fatal diseases, also, given enough time, are taken for granted by those suffering from them.

Medical illnesses are not worrisome for very long to most people even when those illnesses are serious. Strong feelings and the thoughts that accompany them fade over time when nothing obvious is happening. If the danger never gets closer, we tend to forget about it. When heart disease threatens, we are supposed to appreciate the danger sufficiently to take those well known measures that lower the risk, but in the face of month after month, and year after year of nothing happening - no symptoms-or no <u>new</u> symptoms at any rate - even those who know themselves to be vulnerable will become neglectful. If no immediate action is required, the feeling of being sick and the corresponding thoughts fade away.

Even someone who has already had a heart attack will likely put the risk of another out of mind if enough time passes without incident. People get used to their symptoms if they are not getting worse. Similarly, someone who has cancer that has already spread may know very well that he or she is likely to die of that illness but, nevertheless, not worry if no new lesions have developed. No one thinks of death as imminent. Even someone in the hospital with a terminal illness does not know if he or she will die tomorrow or a month from now and, in the absence of some acute symptoms, such as pain, will go back to worrying about some other matters or not worry at all.

Health worriers are different. For the reasons described in the previous chapters, they can keep worrying in the face of no particular danger.

Some points to keep in mind about physical illness.

Most of the important illnesses that doctors spend their professional lives studying and treating are chronic. They do not go away entirely when treated successfully. They are lessened in severity, perhaps, or they may become intermittent. When someone sick comes to their offices, those are the illnesses they consider and rule out. *Undoubtedly, there are many other unnamed, even unknown, illnesses which come and go quickly and for that reason never get described in medical textbooks.* They cannot be explained by the doctor because they are not truly understood. Any explanation of their symptoms manufactured by the doctor will be offered only as a way of telling the patient not to worry.

People not inclined to worry about their health know that most of the time physical problems will disappear on their own sooner or later; so they typically postpone going to the doctor. The disadvantages of putting off going to a doctor are two:

1. Some illnesses will go away more quickly if they are treated promptly. A number of infectious diseases fall into this category.
2. A few grave illnesses such as a heart attack cannot be treated well and may even be dangerous if not treated promptly.

The advantages of not rushing to a doctor are these:

1. The great majority of acute illnesses do, indeed, get better without treatment. Many others will respond just as well if treatment is postponed for a while - for example, irritable bowel syndrome or acid indigestion.
2. Medical illnesses do not develop characteristic symptoms all at once. Diagnosis is difficult when the patient presents with only vague and nonspecific complaints. A person whose only symptom is fatigue could have any sort of physical or emotional disorder. The same person a few days later may have developed a rash or a localizing pain or some other sign or symptom strongly suggestive of a particular illness.

The difficult role of the patient is to determine whether his or her current symptoms suggest one of those rare times when medical consultation should be sought urgently or whether a visit to the doctor can be safely postponed and often avoided.

Chapter Five: Doctors and How They Think

The Role of the Doctor

Question: Can I trust my doctor?
Answer: It depends.
Questions: Can I believe everything he tells me?
Answer: No.

The typical board-certified physician is exceedingly well-trained. As likely as not, he or she was a science major in college, underwent four years of medical school, 3-5 years of residency training, and often years of practice which included further required reading, conferences and other special experiences. Probably no other profession requires as much knowledge. Another kind of knowledge grows out of daily interaction with sick people, all of whom are distinctive, since the same illness presents differently in different people. A doctor is truly an expert. Are experts all equally expert? No. In fact, some experts turn out not to be competent, or conscientious. Is someone who is truly expert always right? Of course not. Should you trust your life to an expert?

In small matters it is reasonable to expect any trained person to do a job satisfactorily. Any plumber can be called for a malfunctioning toilet.   But if pipes begin to leak behind a wall, or if a suggested repair is said to cost three zillion dollars, it is good to get a second opinion. Any doctor can be relied on (trusted) to handle commonplace problems. If a serious illness is thought to be present, however, it is sensible to go to a specialist. When that illness does not respond to treatment, it is reasonable to get a second opinion although not a third, fourth, and fifth. Some medical conditions are very rare and should be seen by an authority in the field. Some surgical procedures are so serious it is reasonable to go to a specialized medical center where that procedure, however uncommon otherwise, is dealt with frequently. Complicated gastrointestinal surgery has fewer complications when done in centers that specialize in it.

When a patient of mine was told he needed to have part of his heart and aorta removed, I thought he was sensible to consult with all three of the cardiac surgeons that were known for that operation even though they were in different parts of the country. In short, the decision on whether or not to rely on your doctor should not depend on your judgment about his or her competence, because that is hard for a lay person to determine, but rather on the nature of the medical problem. But health worriers, it seems, <u>always</u> have trouble trusting their doctors.

When Blanche was in her mid-thirties, she had urinary problems that extended over a period of a few months. These cleared with treatment, but her urologist thought there was reason to perform cystoscopy, which allowed him to visualize the bladder mucosa directly. After the procedure, he told her that she was fine, but to call later in the week to find out the results of the routine biopsies he had taken. When she did call, he informed her with some embarrassment that the biopsies had been lost. However, he assured her unequivocally that he could see her entire bladder, and that she was fine. The biopsies were simply standard procedure and would not have come back positive in any case. She no longer had any symptoms; and she forgot about the incident.

Ten years later, her mother became ill with breast cancer; and, for no particular reason, Blanche found herself thinking about the lost biopsies. She called her urologist, who said again that she had no reason to worry. For one thing, she had been fine over the intervening 10 years. When he found that she was worried still, he told her to come to his office. He spoke to her there at length but could see that she was still concerned that, like her mother, she could have cancer. Perhaps because he felt guilty over the missing biopsies, or simply to reassure her once and for all, he scheduled another cystoscopy.

Afterwards, when he left the procedure room, he said to her something doctors do not usually say. " You're perfect," he told her.

"But I get funny feelings in my bladder sometimes. Why do I get funny feelings?"

"I don't know; but you're perfect."

He spoke to her pleasantly for a few moments and then left to examine another patient. On the way out Blanche saw him across a hallway and waved goodbye.

"Good luck," the doctor called after her.

She left the office and began thinking, "why did he find it necessary to wish me good luck?" She wondered if there was some reason to be concerned.

She came back into the office and asked the doctor why he had wished her good luck.

"I didn't wish you good luck," he replied.

She left again, wondering why he now denied making that remark.

She began to worry that, perhaps, the doctor was keeping something from her. Recognizing that perhaps she was being irrational, she made an appointment to see her psychiatrist, whom she had also not seen for many years. The two of them spent the session agreeing, he thought, that, of course, there was no conceivable reason to worry about her bladder. They laughed together. When she left, he wished her a good summer.

She returned almost at once. "What did you mean by that?" she asked with a worried expression.

It seems remarkable that an intelligent person who is not very sick should seek reassurance from a competent doctor who is trying very hard to be reassuring, and yet fail to be reassured! Often, despite the doctor's best efforts, the patient comes away feeling misunderstood and shunted aside. If the patient feels threatened by a serious illness, he or she will feel specially frustrated and resentful.

In part, the difficulty stems from a misunderstanding on the part of patients of the way doctors are trained to think. Health worriers look for a kind of information that doctors do not have. They ask the wrong questions and consequently get misleading answers. Doctors are not interested in what causes a particular symptom except insofar as that information provides a clue to a particular disease process and, more important, to what needs to be done to make the patient better. In a very real sense, the basic first causes of most illnesses are usually not known. Even in those cases when a disease has an infectious cause, the exact manner in which that agent works is usually unknown.

For instance, AIDS, 20 years after it was first reported in the medical literature, is believed by most, but not all, to be caused by the HIV virus. Some experts think another virus, or other co-factors such as environmental factors, must be present for the illness to develop. No one is sure how these purported cofactors work. It is suspected that some people are genetically invulnerable to the virus. No one knows why. One of the common presenting symptoms is a form of skin cancer called Kaposi's sarcoma. No one knows exactly how the AIDS virus causes it to develop. Full-blown AIDS develops anywhere from a few years to 12 or 13 years following infection. No one knows why some people get sicker earlier than others. Some people get certain secondary infections, and others do not. No one knows why. No one knows why certain people get a dementia from the virus and why others do not. There may be other influences such as autoimmunity or vitamin deficiencies that cause one or another feature of the illness. No one understands how. And so on. And at this point AIDS is as well-studied as any infectious disease in history. I could have described leprosy, which is an ancient disease and is understood no better.

The autoimmune diseases and the degenerative diseases, including cancer, and every other kind of disease, produce their effects in ways that are, in the final analysis, largely unknown. Diabetes, which affects very many people and which has been studied as far back as Hippocrates, is still mysterious. Only in the last few years have we learned that peptic ulcers, thought previously to be a psychosomatic disease, are caused in part by Helicobacter pylori, a commonplace bacterium. Of course, no one knows how the infection is communicated or why some people who are infected get ulcers and others do not. So, when the health worrier asks, "why am I coughing? And, why did I get sick just at this particular time?" he is asking existential questions on the order of "Why me?" or "How did I get here?" and is not likely to get a sensible answer. Which is not to say he won't get some kind of answer.

Patient: "Doc, what is this rash?"

Doctor: (A tall, distinguished-looking internist, wearing a white coat): "It's a neurodermatitis," (meaning this rash looks like the rash labeled neurodermatitis in the dermatology textbook, and also like the rash on that kid the dermatologist showed everyone last week, and also like the 15 or 20 rashes that I've called neurodermatitis over the years. Also, it's in the right location and it itches.)

Patient: What's a neurodermatitis?

Doctor: It's just a rash. Put on this cream three times a day and try not to scratch it.

Patient: Yeah, but what is it?

Doctor: It's ... a non-specific rash. Has an allergic component, probably.

Patient: Allergic? What am I allergic to?

Doctor: Could be anything. Something you wash with. Maybe something you're eating. It should go away with the cream.

Patient: I'm not eating anything new. I'd like to know if I'm allergic to something.

Doctor: Well, I could send you to an allergist; but, you know, they'll test you and it'll turn out you're allergic to a dozen things, like everybody else. If you use this cream, it'll probably just go away. You remember, you had a rash like this before, and it went away with a cortisone ointment.

Patient: That rash looked a little different to me. And it was over here on the other arm. What do you mean, "probably go away." What happens if it doesn't go away?

Doctor (frowning): It doesn't matter which arm the rash is on. If this cream doesn't work, I'll give you something stronger.

Patient: Last time you gave me an ointment.

Doctor: Doesn't matter. Ointments are a little greasier. You can have an ointment if you want. Or a cream. Whatever.

Patient: Why now, do you think?

Doctor: Why now what?

Patient: I mean, why does a rash like this come on out of the blue?

Doctor (shrugging): Why does anything happen when it happens?

Patient: Could it be nerves? I've been under a lot of stress recently.

Doctor: Well ... yes. Nerves can make it worse. That's why it is called a neurodermatitis. But if you just take this....

Patient: I'd like to know what it is. I mean, is it an allergy, or is it nerves?

Doctor: Listen,...

Patient: And why does it itch?

Doctor: It comes from scratching. That's what makes it itch.

Patient: You're kidding! It itches first. That's why I scratch it! You know, I have an aunt who just developed some kind of internal cancer, and the doctors said the first sign of it was a rash. Could I have a pancreatic cancer?

Doctor: What? (looking at the rash again) You don't have pancreatic cancer or any other kind of cancer.

Patient: How do you know for sure? I have stomachaches.

Doctor: (beginning to pout): I don't know for sure. If you want, I can run a whole battery of tests, and I still won't know for sure. For all I know, I have pancreatic cancer. The trouble with pancreatic cancer is it develops without any symptoms. Look, what do you want? You want me to send you to an allergist? A dermatologist? What?

Patient: I want to know whether it's due to nerves, or allergies, or scratching it, or what. (touching the rash with a forefinger.) Looks a little like eczema to me...

And so on.

What this doctor knew was that the rash he was looking at was of a type that usually responded to a cortisone cream. Surely, knowing what to do to help a particular medical problem is exactly what most people want and expect from a doctor. Although he might not have said so even to himself, he had only a vague idea about what caused the rash; and had he been a dermatologist, he would have known only a little bit more <u>because not much is known about the ultimate</u> causes of a neurodermatitis or of any other medical condition. Asked by a patient to explain the patient's problem, most doctors will put a name to the condition and give a short description of what that implies. For example: You have some narrowing of the coronary arteries supplying blood to your heart. It's arteriosclerosis. Or, you have hepatitis. That's an inflammation of the liver. Or, you have a bladder infection. Or, you have a strep throat. Or, a bunion. Or, a cataract. And so on. Sometimes the doctor cannot name a disease, but only a symptom. You have tinnitus. Or, you have an irritable bowel syndrome. Or, "chronic fatigue syndrome." Naturally, just naming something does not explain it, but it is true that hearing that one's condition is familiar enough to have a name is somehow reassuring.

I was awakened one morning by my daughter, then 3 years old, crying in the next room. When I went to her, I could see immediately what the trouble was. Her cheek was swollen by a large mass at the angle of her jaw. She had the mumps. And she was very frightened.

"Oh," I said, smiling at her, "you've got a mump."

"Oh, a mump," she repeated, smiling back at me.

She did not know what a mump was; but she was relieved to know that I did.

Experts in every field have their own arcane language to

describe every sort of problem for just this reason. It is a way of pretending to know something; and patients/clients/customers like to know that they are being served by a knowledgeable person. Unfortunately, the inclination to give some sort of answer to every question tends to encourage a kind of blather. Among the questions health worriers ask are:

How did I get sick? Why did I get sick? Why did I get sick now? Why did this happen to me? If this thing made me sick, why didn't it make me sick last time? If this thing made that thing happen, what made this thing happen? And, anyway, how do you know I don't have pancreatic cancer? These questions encourage physicians to rhapsodize. Pressed hard, they tend to give certain replies:

1. Pseudo-technical. "Your rash is characterized by areas of hyperkeratosis. Histologically there may be epidermal spongiosis and a superficial perivascular inflammatory dermal infiltration. That's what causes the itching."

    Is this what the patient wants to know?

2. Vague, off the top of the head babble. "Your problem is due to:
    Allergy and/or
    Stress and/or
    Being run down. And/or
    A virus (There's a lot of this going around) and/or
    Inflammation and/or
    Heredity.

3. True, but unresponsive. "This sort of problem is very common at your age. Often colitis is associated with a stiff back and inflammation of one or both eyes."

    These explanations are not so much wrong as they are beside the point. They are meant to say, "Don't worry. Your illness is ordinary." And that message gets through to most people. But the health worrier listens more carefully. If one doctor says casually "You've probably got a virus," and the next one says "Maybe it's acid indigestion," and a third says "I think it's probably just something you ate," the health worrier concludes that none of them knows what they are talking about. Yet if the doctors consulted among themselves, they would be under the impression that they agreed: their patient had a non-specific gastroenteritis which required no special treatment and which was likely to clear up spontaneously. Health worriers who grab their doctors by the throat in an attempt to squeeze the truth out of them end by hearing medical platitudes, which should not be taken literally. The harder they squeeze, the more fanciful the response. In this respect, doctors resemble other experts: the more specific the information you want, the more they are likely to extemporize.

I am speaking here of good doctors. The health worrier going from doctor to doctor sooner or later runs into bad doctors, who come in different varieties:

1. Standard-type bad doctor (someone who doesn't know as much as he should and has poor judgment, which usually means not being able to tell which medical condition is likely to be present and which others are not.)

A doctor in the habit of diagnosing hypoglycemia told one of his patients that she had this condition despite her having a blood sugar well within the normal range. He recommended that she eat multiple small meals throughout the day. She took this advice literally and made sure she ate something every few hours. Otherwise she became anxious and agitated. In not much time she became preoccupied with her diet.

Her psychiatrist called the doctor to find out how he had arrived at that diagnosis.

"Well," the doctor told him, "I believe that there is such a thing as hypoglycemia," acknowledging that the diagnosis is controversial.

"But her blood sugar is 160."

"Well, what do you want me to do? Send her back, and I'll tell her she doesn't have hypoglycemia."

It did not matter to him what she thought.

2. Agreeable, easily-influenced-type bad doctor. Medicine is a business, and doctors support themselves by pleasing their customers. This consideration weighs too heavily in the minds of some physicians. Confronting an anxious patient, they too readily accede to demands for unwarranted or premature diagnostic procedures, or unnecessary medication, and sometimes even unnecessary operations! Inappropriate diagnostic procedures are not only expensive but may turn up findings that have nothing to do with the patient's illness and, consequently, lead both patient and doctor astray. More tests are done to verify the first tests, leading to more concern and distress.

   The dangers of the inappropriate use of medicine are clear. Drugs are not without risk. It seems sometimes that every time there is a truly devastating drug reaction it has occurred when the drug should not have been given in the first place. For example, the use of antibiotics to treat viral conditions, for which purpose they are ineffective, occasionally causes a very serious overgrowth of pathogenic bacteria in the lower intestine. Sleep medications and laxatives tend to perpetuate the conditions for which they are prescribed. Tranquilizers and pain medications are sometimes given simply to placate patients despite the fact that they are potentially addictive.

   Similarly, some of the investigative procedures that health worriers may talk their way into are not without risk. It is amazing to see how many people have had coronary angiography without having had any symptoms reasonably attributable to heart disease! More upsetting still is trying to help someone cope with the ill effects of an unnecessary surgical procedure. Someone who has been subjected to exploratory abdominal surgery is vulnerable to the development of adhesions which may cause intestinal obstruction and require additional surgery. When such surgery is avoidable in the first place, a bad result is particularly distressing. Surgical procedures to treat chronic pain fail frequently, unfortunately, and may produce painful sequelae of their own.

3. Bad doctors who are uncaring. The health worrier is likely to feel every other doctor is of this type; but the fact is that they are few. But they do exist.

　　A doctor was called away from lunch to answer the telephone. Only his end of the conversation could be overheard.

　　"Yeah, well ... come on into the hospital. We'll admit you ... You don't want to? ... Well, what do you want? You want a tranquilizer?"

　　What is going on here? What condition requires hospitalization, but when hospitalization is not done can be treated just as well with a tranquilizer? If hospitalization is really indicated, with all that entails, should not the doctor make an attempt to convince the patient? Every patient is entitled to the doctor's time and effort, and health worriers, who require more, are entitled to more. The proper management of the delicate relationship of the health worrier to his or her doctor is central to treatment. This is discussed in the chapters on treatment.

4. Bad doctors who have a particular hobby-horse to ride or who have particular blind spots.

　　A doctor advertised himself as an expert on chronic lyme disease. He claimed to have diagnosed and treated hundreds of cases, including very many that had failed previously to be diagnosed by other physicians. In other words, he was prepared to call something lyme disease when other doctors were not. In his opinion, anyone with muscular pains and a history of a positive lyme test was suffering from chronic lyme disease. Consequently, a number of his patients who really had rheumatoid or osteoarthritis received a useless course of intravenous antibiotics and went without proper treatment.

　　Another doctor considered panic disorder, attention deficit disorder and stuttering all to be manifestations of the same inner ear problem. Similarly, some doctors focus on temporal mandibular joint problems, which they think can cause anxiety, depression and a half-dozen other symptoms. Doctors who specialize in chronic fatigue syndrome are sometimes blind to all the other conditions that can cause fatigue.

Patients who feel dissatisfied with their medical care, among whom health worriers are over-represented, may sooner or later find themselves in the offices of fringe medical practitioners. Some examples: doctors whose first reaction to hearing a physical complaint is to do an analysis of hair or nail clippings for heavy metal poisoning; nutritionists who are able to explain any symptom in terms not only of low blood or tissue levels of certain nutrients, but in terms of the ratios of those nutrients; and toxicologist-allergists who conclude usually that the patient is suffering from an intolerance to all the chemical detritus of our civilization, including such things as newsprint, and who recommend in severe cases living far away in the desert in a plastic room.

There are doctors who recommend for every ailment one or another preferred regimen, perhaps "blood cleansing" or "proper breathing" exercises. And this leaves out many other therapists who operate, one might say, on the other side of the fringe. These include specialized massage therapists of different sorts and iridologists, who are able to diagnose systemic disease by studying the location of spots on the iris of the eye. And, of course, there are psychic healers of many persuasions. Many of these practitioners seem to end up in California for some reason.

Among those doctors who have blind spots are those who take no interest in whether or not a patient smokes cigarettes, a huge health hazard that causes and complicates many medical conditions. Other doctors are too demure to ask about sexual functioning, which is important not only in its own right but because it may be a manifestation of an otherwise obscure disease process or of a drug side-effect. Some doctors will not take note of an emotional disorder. They feel uncomfortable referring patients to a psychiatrist, and they are not prepared to treat them themselves. Even without a great deal of formal psychiatric training, the average family doctor who is knowledgeable about drugs and is willing to meet with patients from time to time can treat certain serious and common conditions, such as depression. This is an illness that may come to the family doctor's attention first because it causes physical symptoms. Health authorities have conjectured recently that one fourth of all clinical depressions go undetected and untreated.

5. Bad doctors who are interested primarily in making a lot of money.

In a lifetime of medical practice, I doubt if I have met, or even heard of, more than 2 or 3 doctors who would knowingly put a patient through unnecessary laboratory investigations or medical procedures just to make money. Unfortunately, doctors are influenced, I think unconsciously, by a more subtle consideration: The Proper Workup. Doctors who understand that the patient almost certainly has a condition which they can diagnose with still greater certainty by, let's say, passing a tube, a procedure for which they will be paid $500, are easily convinced to pass that tube. Similarly, some gynecologists perform hysterectomies in circumstances that the rest of the profession has determined do not require that operation. There are other procedures and tests that can be performed by doctors who are similarly "conservative" (meaning extra careful). And doctors may see patients in general a little more frequently than absolutely necessary "in order to be sure." Hospitals are so financially hard pressed these days that there are subtle pressures on doctors to admit patients to keep bed utilization at 100% of capacity (or more); and this consideration may influence doctors. At the same time because of pressure from cost-conscious government authorities and managed care companies, doctors may be encouraged to discharge patients prematurely for financial reasons.

The fact that doctors are sensible to the possibility of being sued for malpractice provides another incentive to do everything imaginable relevant to the diagnosis of a particular malady. Trying to nail down a diagnosis in this way is usually unnecessary since in most cases time will inform the doctor of the correctness of his or her initial judgment. There is room for error. The patient's ultimate recovery is not usually threatened by the doctor making the wrong diagnosis tentatively - first of all because most conditions improve on their own and go away eventually; secondly, because a condition that is misdiagnosed and even mistreated originally will rarely worsen quickly past the point where the diagnosis can be reviewed safely and a different treatment instituted. In other cases, still more rarely, the timing of the diagnosis is not important because the condition will not be responsive to treatment anyway. This is not an argument, of course, for being careless the first time around; but it is an argument for proceeding at a proper pace. Good doctors will not be hurried into performing every sort of diagnostic maneuver. They understand that there is a cost to be paid by patients, particularly a psychological cost, and a cost that is particularly heavy for those who worry excessively about their health in the first place.

Some of these costs have been mentioned above in general terms; but there is a day to day cost.

Claire was a childless woman of 48 who had recently lost a brother and mother to cancer. She had been in psychotherapy for a social phobia, a kind of exaggerated self-consciousness, but had never worried about her health. In fact, she had always been in good health. However, on one Christmas, not long after the death of her family members, she developed a cough and a low-grade fever. Her condition was diagnosed as bronchitis, and she responded promptly to antibiotics. She was well when she returned to her doctor; but, perhaps because she had been made uneasy by the cancer in her family, she requested an x-ray. The doctor did not think it was necessary since she had had an x-ray the previous year and every few years before that. She had never smoked cigarettes or had lived with anyone who smoked. But he agreed.

The x-ray was read as normal, but "streaky." Reviewing the old x-rays, the radiologist thought these too might be "streaky." He said it might be useful to order a CAT scan of the chest, which Claire's doctor acquiesced to with no great enthusiasm. First of all, Claire was not sick. And lung cancer, he explained, was rare in non-smoking women. Still, he admitted he could not be certain she did not have cancer. So they scheduled the test. The CAT scan showed a number of "patchy," perhaps nodular, lesions in the lower right lobe of the lung. Over the next few months, during which Claire was anxious all the time, sometimes to the point of crying, she underwent a number of medical tests to explain the CAT scan findings. These included a positron-emission scan (PET scan) which, unfortunately, was unable to tell definitively whether the lesions in her lung were active or not. The radiologist thought she could have granulomatous nodules caused, perhaps, by fungal infections or old tuberculosis. She had always had a positive tuberculin skin test. She had a skin test for sarcoid, a poorly understood inflammatory condition which, like many other medical conditions, could be serious, but is usually not. The test was read as equivocal. She had samples of her blood sent away to look for certain very unlikely infectious illnesses. These were negative. Repeated CAT scans showed no change, except for the last one which one radiologist thought demonstrated a subtle enlargement of one of the nodules. Another radiologist did not agree. Cancer was still a possibility, although still unlikely.

Claire's physicians, now three in number, agreed that a lung biopsy should be performed. Somehow, in a complication of the procedure that is not supposed to happen, the biopsy caused a collapsed lung. Claire was hospitalized for a number of days and underwent various procedures to re-inflate the lung. The biopsy had not returned any abnormal tissue. And so matters rested. Claire never got sick with anything; but it was many months before she stopped being afraid that she had lung cancer.

The general level of health anxiety - what could be called

health anguish in some cases - would be lower if unnecessary tests could be avoided. Yet some doctors often find reason to order every test possible.

Perhaps it is easier to spot the infrequent bad doctor in other ways:

A bad doctor is someone who:

1. Does not listen carefully to the patient's concerns.
2. Jumps to conclusions - often to the same conclusion with different patients.
3. Is condescending and smug or authoritarian in manner. Arrogant, it seems to me, is not so bad. Someone who prides himself or herself on knowing more than everyone else is likely to be well informed.
4. Has little interest in the patient's life apart from the patient's illness.
5. Is hard to reach by telephone.
6. Is rushed or disorganized or invariably late.
7. Does not bother to find out how the patient is responding to treatment, even when the patient is seriously ill.
8. Does not bother to call the patient promptly with the results of laboratory tests.
9. Orders unnecessary tests to escape having to rely on his or her clinical judgment.
10. Offers no explanation of the patient's illness or of the reasons for treatment. Or offers glib and careless explanations.
11. Does not have time to speak to the patient's family.
12. Becomes angry if the patient, because of a lack of information, hesitates to undergo recommended tests or take prescribed medications.
13. Never takes into consideration specific and treatable emotional disorders, such as depression.
14. Is inclined frequently to diagnose a favorite disease on which he regards himself as an expert, for example, heavy metal poisoning

or chronic lyme disease or chemical insensitivity.

15. Does not keep up with the medical literature.
16. Uses meaningless terms such as "holistic" as a way of making his services seem special.
17. Pretends to be sure when he is not.

A good doctor is harder to define. It is desirable that a physician should be a decent person who cares about his, or her, patients, who is attentive, interested, reachable, and scrupulous, and willing to spend time also with families, and diligent about making sure the treatment works. It is nice to have a doctor with a good bed-side manner; but what is critical is that he or she has clinical judgment. Clinical judgment is a subtle quality of mind that is hard to measure. Good doctors with good clinical judgment know they have it. Bad ones do not know they do not have it.

Let me describe how doctors are trained to think. A patient comes through the door and the doctor notices things, somewhat as Sherlock Holmes, who was modeled after a physician, might. What the doctor sees looking at the patient is various shades of ordinary: someone of a particular age and sex and race, dressed in a certain way, of a particular posture, erect or bent over, walking, perhaps, with a gait that is normal or stiff and slowed, or mincing, or unsteady, making gestures that are coordinated or not, with a complexion of good color or not, of firm voice or not. Most important: a patient's facial expression reveals a lot. Is that person depressed? In pain? Frightened? All of these observations narrow the possibilities of the patient's illness. Doctors often talk among themselves about a patient simply "looking sick." It is a remark that is always taken seriously.

The doctor then focuses on the patient's chief complaint. This is the patient's principle symptom and its duration.
"I have a bad pain in my back which shoots into my groin."
"I've been getting these splitting headaches that make me throw up."
"I cough all night".

"I see streaks of blood in my bowels".

"My vision is blurry".

"I'm so tired, I have to push myself up the stairs."

Of the various symptoms that drive someone to consult a physician, fatigue is the most common.

The chief complaint further constrains the number of possible illnesses the patient may have. Instead of a world of possibilities, the doctor is searching on only a single continent. Perhaps a half-dozen illnesses, or at least groups of related illnesses, come to mind.

The <u>history of the present illness</u> is an account partly in response to the doctor's questions of how the patient's symptoms began and how they evolved. Often the patient does not know what is relevant, but the doctor does. Since each disease has its own characteristic story-starting a certain way, progressing over a particular length of time to include certain typical symptoms - the doctor finds himself matching up the patient's story to the story of one or another disease. Everything the patient says divides the continent of all possible diseases into countries, then into states and provinces. The doctor does not ask any old question that comes to mind, but only those that pertain to a particular set of medical disorders that he or she already has in mind. How good a history the doctor takes depends on his overall knowledge of medicine. It is often said that a good doctor can usually come to a proper diagnosis 90% of the time prior to doing a physical examination.

Still prior to that examination, the doctor does a: <u>Review of Systems</u>, which is a series of routine questions about the various organ systems of the body, such as the heart or the urinary track. They are intended to uncover problems that the patient may not have thought to mention or the doctor to ask about. They may suggest the presence of an entirely different illness that may have nothing to do with the patient's current complaints. Finally, this sort of ancillary information bears on therapeutic decisions. For example, a medicine that might ordinarily be used to treat a joint inflammation might be contraindicated if the patient is also suffering from asthma.

To complete the history, the doctor asks questions about <u>Past Medical Illnesses, Personal History</u> and the <u>Family History</u> since these too bear on diagnosis.

The <u>Physical Examination</u> is directed by the history. A good physical is not necessarily one that takes forever or includes everything. It is an attempt to discover specific and relevant facts. It is not an exhaustive attempt to look at everything in the body, inside and out, in a manner somehow like a cleaning service might attack a suite of offices. It is more like an explorer trying to follow a path drawn faintly on a map. Having taken a good history, the doctor knows more or less where to go to look for confirming signs. If the patient's chief complaint is a sore throat, it is reasonable to pay more attention to the examination of the throat and neck than, let's say, to the fingernails. If the patient comes to the doctor's office with painful and deformed fingernails, on the other hand, it would be reasonable to spend more time looking at the fingernails than at the throat. What is less obvious is the fact that a good clinician suspecting a lung cancer would still spend some time looking at the fingernails since, for reasons that are not well understood, as usual, lung cancer may cause a swelling of the fingertips called clubbing.

A good physical examination, like a good medical history, depends on the doctor's knowledge and judgment, not solely on a willingness to spend enough time and effort to look into every bodily crevice. Although every physical examination includes routine observations of all the different organ systems-just as a good medical history includes a routine review of systems - the measure of a good physical examination is its ability to discern relevant information. Doctors do not just look around, they are looking for something in particular:

At the end of this process the doctor is obligated to make a conjecture about the patient's illness: a <u>diagnosis</u>. Taking into consideration the patient's complaints and physical signs, the diagnosis is the most likely explanation. It is, as it were, a statistical statement. It is rarely certain. Often the doctor will mark down on the patient's chart a number of other possibilities too. "Rule out" this condition-or the other. "Rule out" means make sure, if possible, with laboratory procedures or further examination, that these other possible, although less likely diseases, are not present. In principle one can go on indefinitely ruling out more and more unlikely conditions; but it turns out the correct diagnosis is usually a common illness. If a patient has a rash, one thinks of eczema or a neurodermatitis before one thinks of leprosy.

In short, a good physical examination depends on the doctor having a good understanding of all the possible illnesses that could explain the patient's symptoms. This is one aspect of good clinical judgment. If the doctor does not consider certain unusual illnesses, there is no chance that he will look for those signs that will make the diagnosis. A good doctor will think of all such possible illnesses, but will not necessarily give them equal weight.

Horses vs. zebras vs. unicorns

There is an old saying in medicine that every student learns in medical school: "When you hear the sound of hooves, think of horses, not zebras." In other words, think of the common diseases, not those that are rare. It is proper, though, to think both of horses and zebras. Still, the correct diagnosis is likely to be that of a common illness; and proper treatment, of course, depends on the proper diagnosis. For example, a simple diarrhea coming on suddenly is likely to have an infectious course and will respond to anti-spasmodics or, sometimes, antibiotics. But if that diarrhea persists for a few weeks, the doctor must consider less common possibilities such as inflammatory bowel disease. A general rule is to look for more and more obscure illnesses when time and unsuccessful treatment rules out those considered initially.

Health worriers, of course, do not think of the more common

and benign conditions first to explain their symptoms. What jumps to mind is the worst possibility. A simple headache suggests a brain tumor. Chest pain means a heart attack. Any change in bowel habits - not the sort of thing that would be noticed at all by most people - conjures up the threat of colon cancer.

Consequently, they are wrong almost all the time. Not only do they think of zebras whenever they get sick, they think of unicorns.

A woman about 50 years of age became increasingly worried when she noticed her menstrual periods becoming sparse and irregular. She might reasonably have attributed this change to menopause. That would be a horse. An anemia presenting initially as amenorrhea might be a zebra. Or a zorse, something between a zebra and a horse. What she worried about, though, was leukemia because a friend of hers had recently developed leukemia! Leukemia does not become evident with the single symptom of lessened menstrual flow. Leukemia is a unicorn - an impossible explanation.

A middle-aged executive believed that he was developing a heart problem because he had pain in his left foot! He explained, when asked, that he knew heart pain could show up in the left arm, so why not in the left foot. Heart disease is definitely not part of the differential diagnosis of pain in the left foot. A unicorn.

Being able in any particular situation to tell horses from zebras is not easy for a doctor and is a critical element in good clinical judgment. Other facets of clinical judgment include:
• Knowing when to proceed further in investigating a problem (or when to leave it alone with the expectation that the problem will resolve on its own).
• Similarly, knowing when to treat more aggressively and when to give current treatment more time to work.
• Knowing which aspects of the patient's history and physical examination are germane to his or her current complaints and which are coincidental.

Good clinical judgment grows out of book learning and experience and something else which is even harder to define, common sense.

It should be clear from this discussion that a good doctor:
- Does not always arrive at the correct diagnosis right away.
- Does not order as many tests as a bad doctor, but on the other hand may order some that the bad doctor would not.
- Does not always know why the patient became ill at just that particular time that he or she did, and not 2 or 3 years later or 2 or 3 years before.
- Does not always offer medicines when a patient comes in for treatment, since not every illness requires medication.
- Does not always know when the patient will recover.
- Does not always know the exact cause of the patient's symptoms, except, perhaps, that they are not due to certain serious illnesses that may occur to the patient.
- Knows when to refer to someone with more specialized knowledge. A good doctor will <u>never</u> resent a patient, or a patient's family, asking for a second opinion.

If the patient does not get well spontaneously and does not respond to medication, it becomes reasonable to consider increasingly unlikely possibilities. How far to go depends on many factors, including these:

1. How sick the patient is. The sicker the patient, the more urgent it becomes to reach the correct diagnosis.
2. The chronicity of the illness. The longer the illness lasts, the more justification there is for further work-up.
3. Proper timing. Some tests become positive only after an illness has progressed to a certain point. Doing them prematurely will not provide useful information.
4. The dangerousness of particular procedures. Many diagnostic procedures are invasive and carry a risk to the patient. There is an inherent morbidity even in less intrusive tests, including, for

example, stress tests. Certain X-ray studies, such as a barium enema, carry a heavy burden of radiation with all the risk that implies, especially when the test is repeated frequently. Some other studies, like the MRI, are not dangerous, but are certainly uncomfortable; and the patient's comfort is a legitimate medical concern.

5. The availability of proper treatment. Doctors are understandably less aggressive about ruling out diseases which require little or no treatment. One example is mitral valve prolapse, in most cases only an unimportant variation in cardiac structure. Similarly, a doctor may hesitate to test for serious conditions when there is no effective treatment available. Discovering the exact virus that is causing an illness may be only of academic interest for that reason. There are other tests which may not be done because the implication of a positive test is unclear. A new test, the prostatic specific antigen, has neither high sensitivity or specificity. Moreover, no one knows whether the disease the test is designed to look for, prostatic cancer – at least certain kinds of prostatic cancer – should be treated in men over certain age.

6. The expense and inconvenience of further evaluation. It would be nice if medical decisions were made only on a medical basis, but, unfortunately, doctors and patients live in a real world where insurance carriers and other second party payers may or may not choose to reimburse diagnostic procedures. They make sometimes arbitrary determinations of the appropriateness of those tests. Some conditions, such as infertility, may not seem to them to be worth exploring or treating. Often tests are scheduled only after considerable wrangling.

7. Legal implications.

A cardiologist was sued successfully for failing to rule out thyroid disease in a woman with an irregular heart beat. The patient subsequently died suddenly in a "thyroid storm." He announced angrily to his colleagues that from now on <u>everyone</u> he saw would be worked up for thyroid disease.

Doctors routinely order a CAT scan to rule out acoustic neuromas in patients who are dizzy even when they think the chance of someone actually having that tumor is less than one in a thousand.

Doctors have to consider the legal risk to themselves when they omit a test which could, conceivably, diagnose an important illness, however unlikely that illness might be. It is easier to order an expensive test that someone else will pay for than rely on clinical judgment. Often a doctor is pushed to such an expedient by the patient's attitude. A worried, aggressive patient will be subjected to more tests and procedures than is appropriate.

8. Possible distress to the patient. Doctors are sensible to the anxiety patients develop waiting for the results of laboratory tests. If such tests can be avoided possibly by postponing them, doctors will be inclined to do so. Also, some investigative procedures, such as a spinal tap, are physically painful and are put off sometimes until absolutely necessary.

<u>For all these reasons, and more, doctors may choose not to order particular tests at a particular time</u>. Although health worriers naturally wish to know the cause of their symptoms as soon as possible,they should not encourage their doctors to do laboratory tests or procedures that are premature or unnecessary.

At the point when the physician has finished taking a history and performing an initial physical examination, he will also do certain routine laboratory tests on blood and urine, possibly a chest x-ray and, if the patient has passed a certain age, an electrocardiogram. These constitute a tiny fraction of all the laboratory tests he could have ordered. They are screening tests to pick up certain common problems which may not yet have caused obvious symptoms, and which may not be related to the patient's present illness. In addition, he will order those tests that are relevant to the diagnosis of the present illness.

By now the doctor may know what is the matter with his patient, or he may not. He should, however, have a very good idea of the range of possibilities. And he should know what to do next. He should have a plan to take particular steps to make a definite diagnosis, and he may be able, even at this point, to begin treatment. Finally, he will sit down to talk with his patient. It is often at this point that things begin to go wrong between the doctor and the patient who is a health worrier. The health worrier misunderstands the doctor's purposes, asks the wrong questions, and, consequently, gets confusing answers that are unsettling rather than reassuring.

Most doctors subscribe to the modern idea that patients are entitled to know about their illnesses and to participate in treatment decisions when possible. Although good doctors make a conscious effort to explain the patient's symptoms, they often do not do so to the patient's satisfaction for three reasons:

1. They may not themselves understand very well the nature of the disease process, even when the diagnosis is certain and the treatment well known. <u>Fundamentally, no illness is understood completely.</u> It is always possible for a patient to ask questions, therefore, which no doctor, no matter how clever, can answer.

2. To explain all the possible consequences of all the possible conditions a patient may have is to include inevitably very unlikely possibilities that have awful outcomes. A worried patient listening to a long account of this sort tends to focus on the worst possible scenario.

3. Similarly, the more detailed the explanation, the more room there is for misunderstanding. After listening for a while, patients cannot remember what was said; or worse, they remember things that never were said.

Within these constraints, however, doctors will make an attempt to explain what they think the patient's illness is and what they plan to do about it.

It might be instructive to follow two patients with health anxiety up to this point in their medical workup. They are composites of real people. The conversations they had with doctors that I report below are not entirely real, but neither are they fictional. Patients have said such things to me. The symptoms the two of them complain about are common, headaches in one, chest pain in the other. The particular fears they had, of a heart attack in the first case, of a brain tumor in the second, are also common.

Betsy's heart problem.

The setting: A doctor's office, easily recognizable from many television commercials. A bookcase is filled with medical books and journals stacked vertically. There are a number of diplomas hanging on the wall. Behind a neatly organized desk is sitting a middle-aged woman who is also neatly arranged, a clean white coat, black hair pulled back in a bun, a composed expression that seems all at the same time intelligent, interested, concerned and dedicated. It is a practiced expression that comes only after some years of experience. Sitting in front of her at the edge of her chair is Betsy, a 27 year old slightly chubby, well-dressed woman.

Doctor (smiling): Well, your EKG is normal. So are the X-rays. The laboratory results look okay so far too. I don't think you have anything to worry about from the chest pain you've been having.

Betsy: Well, what's causing the pain?

Doctor: It's probably just acid indigestion. Heartburn.

Betsy: No ... I don't know. This wasn't really burning. It was a real pain. Right in the center. That's where cardiac pain is supposed to be isn't it?

Doctor: Yes, it is. But that's where the esophagus is too. You see, sometimes the cardiac valve on the stomach goes into spasm-that's just the muscle on the top of the stomach. It has nothing to do with the heart-and then you can get pain. Real pain. Or you can get reflux. We call it GERD, gastroesophageal reflux disorder. The stomach acid gets into the esophagus where the mucosa isn't equipped to deal with it, and you get burning.

Betsy: Pain, not burning … it feels like.

Doctor: Right, pain. You get pain.

Betsy: You said "probably." You're not sure?

This is a bad question. People with health anxiety like to be sure, just as compulsive people in general do; but in that strict sense, it is not possible to be absolutely sure. Just as someone cannot know for certain that he turned off the stove this morning, he cannot know for certain that a particular pain is due to a particular cause. Outside of mathematics, nothing is certain.

Doctor: (still smiling): Well, I'm pretty sure. Chest pain at your age is usually due to esophageal dysfunction of some sort – which is no big deal. Or it comes from the chest wall. If your chest had been tender when I pressed on it, or if the pain got worse when you moved, I would say maybe it was due to a muscle sprain, but as it is, I think it's due to ordinary indigestion.

Betsy: You just said reflux … GERD.

Doctor: Right. GERD. Heartburn. It's all indigestion more or less.

Betsy: What causes it?

Doctor: Well, it depends. Some drugs make the stomach sphincter open up when it shouldn't. Certain foods. You should stay away from alcohol and spices and chocolate. It's a good idea not to eat anything before going to bed.

Betsy: I haven't been taking any drugs.

Doctor: It doesn't have to be drugs. Even stress can do it.

Betsy: Stress? Why? How does stress do it?

Another bad question. A patient may ask why she has particular symptoms and even ask how the condition she is said to have may cause those symptoms, but when she asks why the illness causes those symptoms, she is starting down an endless chain of whys in which the doctor has to admit ignorance sooner or later. Or, worse, make up an answer. So much is true of any question about the world.

Little boy: Daddy, why is the weather hot?

Daddy: Because it's summer. When it's summer, it gets hot.

Little boy: Why, daddy?

Daddy: (Who happens to be a scientist): Because the earth is tilted on its axis. I mean, it's tilted like this ball here. When the top part is tilted closer to the sun, then it's summer. The sun makes it hot.

Little boy: How does the sun make it hot?

Daddy: Well ... the sun has a lot of stuff .. Hydrogen. Radiation. You see, it's a kind of gas. When it turns to helium because gravity squeezes it, it gets very hot. And that makes the sun hot.

Little boy: What makes gravity squeeze the gas, Daddy?

Daddy: Heh, heh. That's really a good question. When there's a lot of mass... When something is very big like the earth or like the sun which is even bigger, then gravity squeezes things together.

Little boy: How does it do that?

Daddy: Here, take the ball and play with that boy over there.

It takes only a very few questions to press anyone beyond the point of being able to explain anything.

Doctor: Stress seems to make it worse. You can tense up any part of the body and get pain.

Betsy: It came the first time after I ran up a couple of flights of stairs. My heart started to go like mad.

Betsy wants to make sure the doctor knows all the relevant details even though she herself does not know what is relevant. She does not trust the doctor to ask the right questions.

Doctor (smiling): Well, if you run up a couple of flights of stairs, your heart is supposed to go fast.

Betsy: How do you know this isn't a case of a missing coronary artery, like that basketball player who dropped dead suddenly?

A very bad question, hard to answer sensibly. These conditions are entirely different. How do I know I'm eating a roast turkey and not a large fish? Well, a turkey is the right size to fit on a platter. It's surrounded by gravy and cranberries, which are associated with roast turkey more frequently than with fish. It's Thanksgiving, which is an important clue. In short, on the basis of my professional judgment, what I think I have in front of me is a turkey.

Doctor: You have no sign of heart disease.

Betsy: Neither did that basketball player...

Doctor: I'm going to give you some medicine for the stomachache...

Betsy: I mean, how do you really know I didn't have a heart attack?

Doctor (sighing): Well, for one thing, there is the quality of the pain. A heart attack typically produces a severe, crushing chest pain which persists...

Betsy: My pharmacist told me you can get a heart attack with just mild pain or even no pain.

Mentioning the pharmacist is probably a mistake. Doctors as a group do not think pharmacists are competent to give medical advice, especially when they have not taken a detailed medical history or performed a physical examination as the doctor just did.

Doctor(a note of impatience creeping into her voice): Yes, that's true. But a heart attack *usually* causes severe pain. People who have had heart attacks look sick. You don't look sick. It's everything all together. You're too young. You're the wrong sex. You have no risk factors for heart disease. Your cholesterol is low. You don't smoke. You have no family history of heart disease...

Betsy: My grandfather died of a heart attack when he was 80. My uncle has angina. And what do you mean I don't look sick? I feel lousy.

Betsy is listening selectively. She is not asking for the doctor's professional opinion. She is certainly not weighing the pros and cons of a particular diagnosis as the doctor is trying to do. Whether she realizes it or not, she is looking for evidence to support a preconceived idea: that she has heart disease. The more the doctor says, the more likely it is she will find something to support that idea.

Doctor: Having a grandfather who dies at 80 of a heart attack *is not* what is meant by a family history.

Betsy:　My grandmother was supposed to have angina too.

Betsy is making another mistake here, and it is the single most characteristic error made by health worriers. She thinks subtle changes in the facts of her life or in the circumstances of her illness are likely to be decisive in determining diagnosis. Later she will report each subtle variation in her symptoms as if each new intricacy will be crucial to the physician's understanding of her case.

"I thought I should call and tell you that the pain came this morning after eating eggs."

"Last night I woke up with the pain, and it was different. It was below my left breast."

"In the middle of the night I woke up panicky. My heart was going a mile a minute, and I felt dizzy too."

Betsy does not know, really cannot know, what is central to understanding her illness and what is peripheral and unimportant. Consequently, she reports everything. And with each revelation she wonders anew, what will the doctor reply? Will she say this time that maybe she is having a heart attack after all?

Doctor (smiling crookedly): You don't have heart disease. *It's my opinion* that you don't have anything the matter with your heart. If this medicine doesn't work, we can always do other tests later on.

Betsy:　You know, I'm really upset. If there are any tests to do, I'd like to do them now.

Here we go. After the first test, there will be other tests. One of the tests will be borderline. The results of another test will be lost, and it will have to be done again. Meanwhile, Betsy will become more and more frantic. Although, typically, health worriers encourage the doctor to order unnecessary tests, it seems just as often they hesitate to take tests the doctor wants to give them because they think the tests themselves might be dangerous.

Doctor: The next test is a stress test. You'd have to spend a few hours here. It's expensive; and it's not necessary! ... All right, I'll schedule a stress test next week if you 're not feeling better by then. Just to be sure.

Betsy: Could it be something else?

Doctor: Could what be something else?

Betsy (annoyed): The pain!

Doctor: It can always be something else! Chest pain can be caused by degenerative diseases, metabolic disease, viruses, tumors, lymphoma, Crohn's disease, gall stones ... A blow to the chest. Did anyone punch you in the chest?

Betsy (stunned and silent for a moment): No.

Doctor (writing a prescription): Good.

Betsy (tentatively): Crone's stones?

Doctor: What?

Both Betsy and the doctor are now confused. Another example of the doctor saying one thing and the patient hearing another.

Doctor (frowning): Have you ever taken any Valium? I'm going to give you a prescription for Valium because I think you're very nervous.

Betsy: Will it help with the pain?

Doctor: (shrugs)

Betsy: You think I'm imagining the pain, don't you?

And so on. Betsy comes away from the interview thinking her doctor is impatient and indifferent. The doctor, it seems to her, is more concerned about the expense of a test than about her peace of mind. She does not believe her doctor is taking her complaints seriously. If the doctor went beyond prescribing a tranquilizer to making a psychiatric referral-which would have been perfectly appropriate since Betsy has an emotional problem which is treatable-she would have been offended further. Betsy also feels confused about the nature of her illness. She heard the doctor mention lymphoma, which she knows is a kind of cancer, so she worries now about that possibility too along with worrying still about heart disease. Despite her doctor's repeated assurances that she is not seriously ill, she is not reassured.

What did Betsy really want to know?

Betsy came to her doctor with real - not imaginary - symptoms. She wanted to know whether her symptoms suggested a serious condition or not; and she wanted to know what to do, or what medicine to take, to make those complaints go away. This is what all patients want when they come sick to their doctors' offices. They have a right to expect that their doctors make medical decisions on the basis of an informed and thoughtful judgment. Some patients expect reasonably to be given an explanation of their condition. Many others have no interest in such an account. *However, those who do want to know about their illness, and why their doctor feels one diagnosis is more likely than another, cannot hope to understand truly why different factors weigh differently in the doctor's mind. First, they would have to be doctors themselves. Diagnosis is a clinical judgment based on years of training and experience.*

What questions should Betsy have asked?

Much of what Betsy wanted to know was explained to her by her doctor on the doctor's own initiative. Betsy, like most patients with health anxiety, was too worried to accept a simple account. Assuming she could not have heard her doctor the first time around, these are questions she might have asked:
1. What do you think is causing my symptoms?

2. What should I do (or what drugs should I take) to make this condition go away?
3. If these measures don't work, what should we do next?
4. Should I be concerned that I might have something more serious, such as heart disease?

Betsy could not find out what she wanted to know because she asked the wrong questions.

Betsy's doctor, and doctors in general, are not altogether blameless in these unsatisfactory encounters. Often, doctors seem to be saying, or doing, something that contradicts what they may have said only a moment before. Betsy's doctor told her a stress test was unnecessary yet only a few minutes later offered to schedule the test. Sometimes the contradiction is not so explicit; but the patients come away from their doctors' offices confused nevertheless.

"They told me in the emergency room that there was nothing physically the matter with me; but then they told me to see my regular doctor the next day. Why? And why did they give me a shot of something if there was nothing the matter?"

"They said I have a benign heart arrhythmia and that I can exercise all I want; so what am I doing here in the cardiac unit?"

"He told me I just have a viral sore throat, so why did he give me an antibiotic which I know doesn't work with viruses?" and "If she thinks there's nothing serious the matter, why did she....

order an M.R.I?"
tell me to stay away from sugar?"
tell me to come back in a month?"
order a barium enema?"
order another barium enema?"
prescribe an anti-depressant?"
ask me to leave when she spoke to my husband?"
send me to a neurologist?"

The answer, of course, is that the doctor is speaking approximately. When she says there is nothing the matter, she is rounding off her answer to the nearest decimal place. Were she to speak exactly, she would be saying, "I'm 96.53% sure you have no serious medical problem, but in order to take no chances, I'm going to order an antibiotic for your sore throat in case it's strep and not really a virus." Or "I'll order another barium enema to reduce the small degree of potential error in the first barium enema." And so on.

Confronting health worriers, doctors try especially to be definite when they express an opinion in an attempt, usually misguided, to be reassuring. And there are some physicians who speak in definite terms as a matter of temperament. In all fairness, though, most patients understand quite well what their doctors mean.

David's brain tumor

It is later the same day. The same physician is sitting behind the same desk. The collar of her white coat is wrinkled and up on one side. A few strands of hair have come down in very slight disarray; but she is still smiling. The afternoon sun is slanting through blinds and falls on a young man sitting in front of her. He is frowning.

David: (We catch him in mid-sentence because he has been talking constantly since sitting down a few minutes ago.) ... day after day, all day it seems, like somebody was squeezing a band around my forehead back around the ears. Over here... sometimes under the ears. Sometimes it's like a cap pressing down around here ... right here, or over here in the jaw. I thought TMJ. My friend is a dentist, he said maybe TMJ. He said I should ask you. You know TMJ? I thought....

Doctor: Temporal-mandibular joint...

David:. problems from that. But the pain is also way over here. I don't see how I can get pain way over here from a joint over here. My friend says you can get dizzy from TMJ problems...

Doctor: No, well...

David: It doesn't throb except hardly at all except sometimes....

103

Doctor: I know, you told me.

David: Right. No flashing lights. No vomiting. I feel a little...I would say... not nauseous, but queasy, maybe. A little unsettled with burping. I don't throw up, but the queasy feeling comes in waves ... little waves with the head pain...sort of queasy.

David thinks that if he could only communicate to the doctor the exact shade of queasiness he gets with his headaches, she would be able to hone right in on the diagnosis.

Doctor: I know. Vascular headaches are usually throbbing. Sometimes only on one side. That's what they mean by "migraine." Migraine causes vomiting. Most headaches are either vascular or tension. You have a typical tension headache.

David: It started when we moved into this new building, so new the windows won't open up. Everyone got headaches and a scratchy throat. So they fixed the windows finally, and now they open; but there's a river right outside and this...this miasma comes up from the river...vapors...and everyone started coughing, but no headaches. I'm the only one who still gets headaches, so I began to worry.

Doctor: Well, it's just a tension headache, I think. If aspirin doesn't work, you can try another anti-inflammatory drug, like ibuprofen. You can also try hot soaks or massage to the neck, or stretching exercises; but, frankly, they don't often help. Tension headaches can recur every day for weeks, even months. Then they go away usually. No one really knows why they come or why they go away. There are other stronger drugs to take later on if the headaches keep bothering you; but they probably won't be necessary.

David: You think?

Doctor: What?

David: You said, you "think." You're not sure?

(Silence)

You're not sure I have tension headaches?

Doctor: No. They're typical tension headaches.

David:　Could they be something else?

Wrong question. Probably there are hundreds of medical ailments that can cause headaches.

Doctor: Well, you know. Anything is possible. But you have typical tension headaches.

David:　What causes them?

Doctor: I just said, no one really knows. Some people think muscular tension in the neck. Maybe emotional tension.

David:　I'm only tense because I'm worried about these headaches.

Doctor: OK.

David:　What about an EEG?

Doctor: No, no. Your neurological examination is negative. An EEG might be helpful to localize a brain tumor or something like that. You don't have to worry about that.

David:　Frankly, I have been worrying about a brain tumor. A friend of a friend of mine just got a brain tumor. He's just my age.

Doctor: You don't have to worry about that. Brain tumors are very uncommon at your age.

David:　Well, it happened to him.

Health worriers - perhaps people in general - tend to argue too much from their personal experiences. We all have a larger number of acquaintances than we realize. All of them have other friends and relatives. It would be surprising if among all these people someone did not have a rare disease!

Doctor: Yes, I know. You just told me.

David:　Could a brain tumor cause a headache like mine?

Definitely the wrong question. What David really wants to ask is: given the fact that I have a headache like the kind I do have, what is the chance of it being due to a brain tumor? The answer to the question he did ask is frightening. Sure, brain tumors may cause a headache like yours. The answer to the question he should have asked is reassuring: Headaches like yours are exceedingly common. Maybe one in 5,000 is due to a brain tumor. This error is made repeatedly in different contexts by health worriers. A man afraid of AIDS develops a sore throat and asks: can AIDS cause a sore throat? Answer: Yes. What he should ask is: since I have a sore throat, what are the chances that it may be due to AIDS? Answer: Nil.

Doctor: Brain tumors can cause any kind of headache. Or none. But you have no sign of a brain tumor.

David: What kind of signs would that be?

Another characteristic error made by health worriers. Most doctors will mention 6 or 7 of their findings that are not consistent with the illness the patient is worrying about - in this case a brain tumor - and the patient will challenge each one, almost as if he or she is trying to find a reason to worry. For example, if the doctor says, you're the wrong age for this illness, the patient asks "aren't there exceptions?" If he says, "This symptom appeared too late to be consistent with that illness," the patient replies, "well, actually I was beginning to feel that symptom a little bit a couple of days before." If the doctor says, "you would have been vomiting, " the patient thinks back and says, "well, I wasn't eating, and I did feel a little sick to my stomach." In the quest for certainty, the patient blurs all meaningful distinctions, sometimes, unfortunately, confusing the doctor also. Patients do not know enough to weigh clinical issues. Checking on the doctor's reasoning is simply not feasible.

Doctor: It wouldn't be helpful to go into that.

David: So what do you think is the matter?

Doctor: (A pause. The doctor stares at David) I think you have a tension headache.

David: Why now? Except for that time a few years ago, I never had headaches.

Bad question. Beside the point. Also, it invites speculation to which David may attach too much significance. Here are some of the usual answers that physicians offer in response to such a question. They provide no useful information.

You have become ill now, probably, because:

1. Your condition is particularly common this season of the year.
2. You have changed your diet.
3. There has been a change of weather (barometric pressure, amount of sunlight, etc.)
4. Of emotional stress.
5. Of physical exhaustion.
6. You caught it from someone: I don't know who, and you can't figure it out.
7. You were sleeping in a funny position.
8. Your age. (Last week you weren't old enough, but this week you are.)

The real answer to "why now?" is "why not now?" Most medical illnesses are present after a period of not being present. Everything had to start at <u>some</u> time. Or to put it differently: the truth is, we do not know why most illnesses begin when they do.

Doctor: (looking out the window and sighing.) I don't know why. It doesn't make any difference.

David: I got a headache yesterday after taking some Vitamin C.

Actually, David got the headache after taking Vitamin C, which he took with his dessert, which was cantaloupe. Loud music was playing at the time, and he had had trouble reading the menu a few minutes before. Also he was eating lunch with his boss. Besides the Vitamin C connection, David is wondering whether his headache was due to sitting with his boss, eye strain, loud noises or an allergy to cantaloupe. It even occurs to him that the headache was in response to something that had happened an hour previously, namely, a car just missing him as he stepped into an intersection. If he were to ask about all these possibilities - and he would like to-he would be in the doctor's office for quite a while; and he has noticed that she has begun fidgeting. Unfortunately, medical illness is too complicated to be explained by whatever circumstances patients may have found themselves in at the moment when they first became symptomatic.

David: (continuing after a momentary silence) I tried foot pressure later on. You know, reflexology, but it didn't help... Do you think I should try bio-feedback.

Doctor: (Riffling papers on her desk.) Sure. It's okay with me. Whatever you want, if you go to a chiropractor, make sure they don't twist your neck too hard. Otherwise... anything.

David: So... what do you think is really the matter?

David has been paying attention more or less. He knows the doctor thinks he has a tension headache; but he wants to know what a tension headache is. He wants to understand his headache is some basic existential sense. He wants to comprehend the fundamental cause, the derivation, the essence of his headache. Actually, he does not know what he wants, but he wants something more. Naturally, the doctor does not understand any of this.

Doctor (voice rising): Look, you have a tension headache. That's all. The chance of your having a brain tumor is maybe one in a thousand. Forget it.

David (upset now): One in a thousand! That much?

This confusion over odds is very common. Obsessional people think one in a thousand is quite a lot. Since overcoming their health anxiety requires that health worriers learn to live by the odds, an important aspect of treatment is teaching them an appreciation, a gut feeling, for what such odds really mean.

David: Isn't it possible to rule out a brain tumor? I'd feel more comfortable if I could be sure.

Doctor: (losing her patience.) All right. Come back in three weeks. If you still have headaches, I'll order an M.R.I. That way we'll be sure. In the meantime I'll order an EEG. Also, in the meantime, I'm going to write you a prescription for a tranquilizer. (She stands up.)

No good. David will not be sure even after the M.R.I. And in the meantime, he is going to worry more than ever. The tranquilizers will not work.

David (feeling rushed) mutters: I hope I'm not going to have this damn headache forever.

This is an interesting idea. Why should David feel that a condition he has had for only a few weeks may go on forever? Although most health worriers have the idea that they may be sick now with a fatal disease, there are others who know that they have only an ear infection or a sore throat and worry nevertheless that they will have these conditions forever, or, at least, on and off forever. Why should they hold to this worry in the face of their doctors telling them otherwise? And why should the thought of having forever a more or less innocuous condition be so upsetting in the first place? In a way, strangely, a similar question can be raised about people who are afraid of having a fatal disease. Since we all know we are going to die, why do some people worry about dying and others do not?

After this interview David returned home thinking that his doctor was impatient and inconsistent. One minute she said an EEG would not be useful, the next minute she ordered one. He was upset that she was so obviously upset with him. Most important, she seemed to him not able to explain his headache. Not to his satisfaction. Despite what she said, he continued to feel there was a definite possibility that he had a brain tumor, or some other condition, perhaps equally serious, that a careful doctor could somehow discover. He had the feeling that somewhere, in some way, there was a laboratory test that could tell him what he wanted to know.

Chapter Six: Laboratory Tests

Patient: Isn't there a test for that disease?

Doctor: There are lots of tests.

Patient: So, why don't we do one of those tests?

Doctor: Because they won't tell us if you have the disease.

One feature of our swiftly advancing medical technology is the rapid development of new, more accurate, medical tests. There are the familiar routine tests of blood and urine and also tests so intricate and difficult they can only be performed in one or two laboratories in the entire country. Doctors can order different tests on blood, urine, feces, saliva and sweat. Every organ can be monitored. There are liver function, kidney function, and pulmonary function tests and tests that measure the subtle interplay of the different endocrine glands. We can measure blood pressure, spinal fluid pressure and ocular pressure. Biopsies are performed routinely on breast, prostate, skin, endometrium and colon and less commonly on liver and kidney, even on brain and heart. Most diseases can be tested for, usually with a variety of tests. AIDS, for instance, has a number of antigen and antibody tests. There are 8 or 9 tests that bear on the diagnosis of systemic lupus erythematosus (SLE). Tubes can be inserted almost everywhere in the body to look for pathological processes. No place is hidden, it seems, from these fiberoptic appliances. The lungs, the heart, the entire colon and the stomach are some of these hitherto unreachable places. The ability of the body to react to peculiar circumstances can be examined. Does someone throw up when ice water is inserted into her ear? Does someone get weak after drinking a sugar solution? Does someone develop a cardiac arrhythmia when a special electrical probe is passed into the heart with the specific intent of causing the arrhythmia if possible? It is hard to believe that there is some organ so cleverly hidden in the body that it cannot be successfully prodded and probed.

Most extraordinary of all are new machines that can visualize the internal structure of the body without entering it. Bones and various other organs can be scanned using radioactive markers. Ultrasound, a kind of radar, is used routinely to inspect the gall bladder, the liver, the bladder and many other soft tissues. Even the hard container of the skull can be penetrated by x-rays which can be summed up and manipulated by computer to depict any desired cross-section. The same structures seen through magnetic resonance imaging (MRI) show different kinds of pathology.

These laboratory tests are truly wonderful. They provide a new dimension to the practice of medicine. Neurologists used to pride themselves on being able on the basis of an examination of the patient to pinpoint the exact area of the brain which had been affected by a tumor or a stroke. Nowadays they can get the same information by looking at a series of pictures. Expensive pictures.

Sometimes the information garnered by these tests is critical and obtainable in no other way. There are other times, through, when these tests are ordered "for the record."

A man visited an otolaryngologist complaining of a sudden onset of vertigo and ringing in the ears. The doctor told him that almost surely he had an acute vestibular (inner ear) problem caused by an infection which would likely go away, treated or not, within a few weeks; but she ordered an M.R.I. of the skull nevertheless. She wanted to make sure, she explained to the referring physician, that the man did not have an acoustic neuroma, which is a benign tumor of the 8th cranial nerve. Although benign, it is a troublesome tumor because it is very difficult to remove after it grows past a certain size. When asked what she thought of the chances of this particular patient actually having this condition, she said no more than one in a thousand! "But how do I explain <u>not</u> ordering the test if the neuroma shows up five years from now?"

"Defensive medicine," such as this, is the systematic attempt to rule out any potentially serious illness <u>no matter how unlikely it may be</u>. These tests are not always done to protect the patient, but rather to defend the doctor against a possible lawsuit for malpractice. Unfortunately, doctors have become wary of their patients. They feel, correctly, that they are likely to be judged by the outcome of their patient's illness rather then by how well they manage it.

There are other times when technology gets used for its own sake. About 20 years ago a man was examined by a cardiologist and told that he had a "benign third heart sound."

"Don't worry," the doctor said, "it doesn't mean anything."

About 10 years later, following another routine examination, the same cardiologist said, "you have a third heart sound, I want to order an echocardiogram in case you have mitral valve prolapse." (The echocardiogram, a device for examining the heart by bouncing sound waves against it, had just been invented.) Mitral valve prolapse is a bend in the way a heart valve closes. The health consequences, in most cases, are trivial.

"You do have mitral valve prolapse," the cardiologist told his patient a few days later after looking at the echocardiogram, "but don't worry, it doesn't mean anything."

"Then why did you want this echocardiogram?" The patient asked.

"Well, it's nice to know definitely."

Technology, particularly new technology, tends to get used simply because it is available. But there are implications to its use.

"Also, the doctor went on, "if you've got mitral valve prolapse, you're supposed to take antibiotics before going to the dentist - to avoid infection on the leaflets of the valve. But don't worry, that's rare," He added, chuckling. "You've got to spend about a million dollars on penicillin to prevent one case of sub-acute bacterial endocarditis."

"So why bother?" The patient asked.

"That's the advice of the hospital lawyer."

Perhaps the lawyer did not take into consideration the fact that some people are allergic to penicillin. They might sue if they had a bad reaction. Maybe lawyers should not be deciding medical practice.

A few years later the same cardiologist looking at the <u>same</u> echocardiogram told the patient that he <u>did not</u> have mitral valve prolapse! "The criteria for making the diagnosis has changed," he explained.

In other words, a diagnosis was sought not because it was thought to be clinically significant, but because the technology was in place to make it. Treatment was recommended not because it was thought to be necessary, but because it was thought to be prudent, marginally, and for legal reasons. And, finally, the diagnosis was dubious. Not uncommonly, performing tests that are not strictly necessary is likely to lead down the road to unforeseen consequences: more testing and, sometimes, treatment with still further unforeseen consequences. This process can continue long after the original complaint has disappeared.

Human beings have a well-developed sense of curiosity. The desire to learn something new is often pursued just for its own sake; and in general this is a good thing. Much of science has this character. But there is always a price to be paid. Vast sums are spent every year on medical testing. Some of this money is spent on research with no direct benefit to patients; but it is money well spent. If the average life can be extended as it has been over the last century, and made healthier, most of us would be prepared to pay the price. When an individual is tested, however, there is a price to be paid in addition to money. A woman told that she should be tested for cancer, however routine that test may be, is likely to worry before the test is taken, during the test, and after, while waiting for the test to be reported back. The more she worries, the more she focuses on her body, and the more inclined she becomes to worry in general about her health.

The Laboratory Test Experience

'Don't worry," the doctor says, "it....
(the lump) or
(the bump) or
(the discharge) or
(the rash) or
(the arrhythmia) is probably nothing, but I want to run a few tests, just in case."
"Call this number, please, and schedule
(an x-ray) or
(an M.R.I.) or
(a biopsy) or
(a stress test) or
(a sonogram) or
(a battery of specialized blood tests) and then call me for the results."

The patient schedules the test at the earliest possible time, which is a week later on Thursday. She telephones her primary physician and explains that she is very nervous having to wait that long, so the doctor calls the testing place and uses his influence to have the test move up to Wednesday.

The patient manages to spend the next few days working and taking care of her children, but she becomes upset at intervals when the examination suddenly looms up in her mind. By Tuesday these inchoate anxieties take up more of the day, and, by Wednesday, they preoccupy her. That night she sleeps badly but arrives promptly the next day for the test, which turns out to be delayed
(a half hour) or
(an hour or so) or
(a day or so) or
(a week) for no clear reason.

Often, when the test is finally administered and the results are known immediately, they are withheld from the patient. It is thought that she may misunderstand the results, the meaning of which differs from patient to patient. Consequently, a nurse will not report them. The primary physician has that responsibility.

The usual practice of a primary physician may be to call patients when laboratory results are reported back, but the worried patient finds waiting for the call too difficult. The worried patient, therefore, is told to call the doctor's office on a particular day. Bright and early that day the patient does call only to be informed that the mail has not arrived yet. Three hours later the patient calls again and is put on hold for approximately a year and a half, it seems. The nurse comes on the line, finally, but tells the patient that only the doctor can speak to her and the doctor will not be in the office until later that afternoon. The patient reasons gloomily that the test must be positive, otherwise, surely, the nurse would have told her the result. When she calls back a third time, the doctor is in the midst of an examination and cannot come to the telephone. The nurse promises he will return the call as soon as possible. For the next hour, the patient stays within 3 feet of the telephone, which does not ring. Finally, at five minutes to five she calls one last time and reaches the doctor's answering service. The doctor's office is closed. He is away for the weekend, but will return early Monday morning.

This scenario is only somewhat exaggerated.

This sort of experience especially troubles health worriers since they start with the expectation that a calamity is always lurking around the comer. Other people think that everything will turn out okay in the end. They do not bother to check to make sure. Health worriers are made worse by waiting around for the latest medical bulletin. It focuses their attention further on their health; and so the habit of worrying gets worse. For this reason medical tests should only be performed for good reasons. That said, health worriers would worry less if they better understood the limitations of all medical testing.

A number of years ago, the 14-year old son of a physician was recovering from an illness that had been serious enough to require hospitalization. His recovery was slow, but otherwise unremarkable. The routine tests he was given at the time included some which were not really routine - probably just because he was the son of a doctor. One of these was the anti-nuclear antibody test (ANA), taken, perhaps, because the patient was anemic slightly, attributable reasonably to his illness, but conceivably due also to a number of other uncommon diseases. The ANA came back positive. This was not really helpful making a diagnosis, though, since it is positive in a wide range of illnesses, including the one he was already known to have. In fact, it is positive in one form or another in a small segment of the healthy. It is positive also, sometimes, in the presence of systemic lupus erythematosus, also called SLE or lupus. This is a serious condition which the treating doctor decided to rule out despite the fact that the patient had none of the wide variety of symptoms and signs that lupus causes. "Just to be on the safe side," he explained. The test thought at that time to be definitive for lupus was the antibody test for double-stranded DNA. This test was performed and was reported days later as "strongly positive," upsetting everyone.

A number of possibilities were considered. The most hopeful, a laboratory error, was ruled out by sending the test to different laboratories, only to be reported back each time still "strongly positive." Certain drugs were known to cause a false positive test, but the young man was taking none of them. The least attractive alternative was that he was in fact in the early stages of lupus; and this was the explanation advanced by a well-known expert on lupus. This is an example of what I call The Expert Syndrome, the tendency of an expert to extend the boundaries of a condition well beyond the usual criteria for making the diagnosis. The textbook definition of lupus requires a number of different symptoms, none of which this young man had. This doctor made the diagnosis of lupus on the basis of this single test alone. Other doctors stated unequivocally that this was not a case of lupus, whatever the test said. And so matters stood for months. Everyone waited and looked anxiously for incipient signs of lupus. And signs of lupus can appear in skin, muscle, joints, nervous system, heart, digestive system and other bodily parts and functions. So there was a lot to worry about. The anemia that had precipitated all this testing and worry had long since gone, but the consequences of the testing persisted.

Three months later, the young man's father came across a very brief reference in a medical journal to a study done on normal blood donors. 5% of normal blood donors had "strongly positive" antibody tests to double-stranded DNA. Two decades later his son had not yet developed any signs of lupus.

Sensitivity and Specificity

No medical test is entirely accurate. First of all, there are the usual mistakes people make in any endeavor. Blood and urine samples get mixed up or lost. X-rays get mislabeled. Slides are misplaced. A sample of blood may stand too long on a shelf with the result that certain values change. The blood sugar level gets lower and lower. One might think that medical matters, which are sometimes life and death, would encourage people to be especially scrupulous; but the fact is everything becomes routine sooner or later and, consequently, people make routine mistakes. Beyond that, however, there is an uncertainty in medical tests that most people do not recognize. The same test performed on a patient and sent off to two different laboratories is likely to come back with two different results. What constitutes normal differs from one laboratory to the next. This correlation is called inter-laboratory reliability. There is also imperfect reliability within a single laboratory. The same blood sample examined by different individuals on different days is likely to give a somewhat different result. The difference may not be significant clinically but is in the range of discrepancy that troubles health worriers.

"Why was my platelet count in the middle of the normal range last week and now it's in the low end?"

Biopsies can be read by one pathologist as high-grade dysplasia, which may be a pre-cancerous condition, and by another as low-grade dysplasia, or as normal. The results may determine the need for major surgery. Medical decisions take this variation into account. <u>Simply repeating a test again does not make it more accurate</u>.

Every medical test has certain systematic limitations which are measurable and which must be understood in order to understand the test.

The <u>sensitivity</u> of a test is the ability of that test to pick up the condition which it was designed to find. No test is 100% sensitive. A mammogram will not show every breast cancer. It will miss a few. An X-ray of an injury will sometimes not demonstrate a fracture that becomes visible, perhaps, only a number of days later. A test on stool for amoebiasis will sometimes be negative when the organism is present. Good tests are often 97 or 98% sensitive. Some tests are useful despite having a lower sensitivity. When a test is correctly positive only half of the time, though, its usefulness is limited. How would someone feel if her pregnancy test came back "no- but maybe yes."

Each test is said also to have a certain <u>specificity</u>, which is the ability of the test when positive to distinguish between the condition the test was designed for and everything else. A test when highly specific will be positive almost always only when that condition is present and not as the result of some other related, or unrelated condition. In other words, specificity is an indication of how often a positive test will turn out to be a true positive or a false positive. The higher the specificity the better the test. If the specificity is too low, the test becomes useless even if the sensitivity is very high. A test reported positive would be like telling the woman mentioned above that her pregnancy test had come back "yes - but maybe no." How helpful is a test for syphilis when the test is positive also in the presence of lupus or a half dozen other conditions? There is such a test.

No test is perfectly sensitive or perfectly specific. It is unusual, therefore, for the diagnosis of an illness to depend on the result of any single test or procedure. Doctors understand this full well, but health worriers do not. They worry much too much over how a test may come out because they exaggerate the amount of information that test conveys. Women would worry less going for a mammogram if they understood that a positive mammogram is more likely than not to be a false positive - and, on the other hand, that a negative mammogram does not rule out the possibility of breast cancer. Often, when a cancer is found, subtle signs of it can be found in previous mammograms that had been read as negative at the time. Nevertheless, it is true that a breast cancer when found initially on a routine mammogram is likely to be curable 95% of the time.

There is still one other oddity of medical testing that confounds interpretation and that is so counter-intuitive, it is hard to believe: two identical tests that turn out exactly the same way can have almost opposite meanings depending on whom the test has been given to!

Let us imagine a very good test for H.I.V., the virus that causes AIDS. This test is 99% sensitive and 99% specific. The most common test is not quite so good, but close. Why not give this test to everyone so that everyone who needs treatment can get it? Certain populations, male homosexuals and I.V. drug users, have a high prevalence of H.I.V.; let's say, for the sake of argument, 10%. The rest of the country has a very low prevalence, about one in a thousand, perhaps. If this test were given to someone in the first two groups, a positive test would be 10 times more likely to be a true positive than a false positive (since only 1% of tests are false positives). Such a person would be told reasonably that it is very likely he has H.I.V. If the same test were given to a person in the general population and came back positive, the result would be 10 times more likely to be a false positive than a true positive! The chance of a true positive is only one in a thousand and the chance of a false positive is still one in a hundred. Such a person would be told, his positive test notwithstanding, that it is very unlikely he has H.I.V. If all such people in the general population were treated, 90% of them would be treated in error! In reality, a more expensive, more difficult, and still more specific test would be used to confirm the diagnosis before starting treatment.

Another example:

A radio-opaque stress test performed on a 49-year old man was considered diagnostic of coronary heart disease. The same test result would not have been regarded as significant if performed on a 20-year old woman. The reason is the same: the frequency of coronary artery disease in middle-aged men is high but very low in young women.

In summary, medical tests deal in probabilities and not certainties. Diagnosis is rarely made on medical tests alone. Changes in these tests may not reflect significant clinical changes. Doctors often speak about treating the patient and not the test. Neither is there a test for every condition. Some parts of the body and bodily functions are still inaccessible.

What, then, are medical tests good for? They tell the doctor what to do next. A positive mammogram may lead to a biopsy which may lead to a curative operation. An abnormality of routine liver or kidney function tests may cause a doctor to suspect diabetes or any of a dozen other conditions and, therefore, look carefully for signs of those illnesses. Sometimes a test can be an indicator of the success of treatment or a reason to try another treatment. Many tests are only vaguely supportive of a diagnosis but taken together with other tests point the physician in a particular direction. Tests can reasonably be considered part of the physical examination. Along with the medical history they usually lead to a proper diagnosis sooner or later - often later. But, they are not "revealed truth." There is no reason to wait for laboratory results with bated breath.

Chapter Seven: Six Principles of Treatment

Health anxiety is an exaggerated fear of physical illness. It is not just a worried state of mind, though, but also an inclination to behave in certain ways. Those behaviors are seemingly designed to calm and reassure, but are driven actually by the need to ward off danger. Since it is an imaginary danger, by definition, the worried state of mind seems to everyone, including the health worrier, to be excessive and irrational. The behavior of the health worrier, serves paradoxically only to sustain that fear. Although irrational, the frantic behavior of the health worrier is, however, a reasonable response to the misconceptions the health worrier has about himself or herself and about the nature of physical illness. These are the Bad Ideas decried in previous chapters. Unfortunately, health worriers cannot take these lessons to heart simply by reading them. They cannot learn how to relax by listening to a lecture. Those who are afraid of flying in airplanes know that it is really a safe way to travel, but they are frightened nevertheless. Those people who are afraid of birds, and there are a number of them, know very well that birds do not usually fly at people; but they are still afraid.

Convictions of this sort are ingrained. They are learned at a gut level and have to be unlearned similarly at a gut level. What does that mean? Health worriers have to test out the world and themselves in such a way that they can see for themselves what is real and what is imaginary. They have to confront their fears systematically in ways that allow of no distortions. Only specific knowledge about one's own body and one's own symptoms can truly reassure the health worrier. The truth is reassuring. Finally, it is only by derailing the worry wheel at various critical points that the individual can feel free and safe enough to turn back to the ordinary concerns of living.

Six principles govern treatment. They are designed to help the health worrier learn the truth insofar as it is possible to know it.
1. Know the truth about yourself; Your particular symptoms, and the

way you react to stress.

Naturally, the physical symptoms that stem from one illness on one occasion, let's say, from a bronchitis, will likely be different from those that occur on another occasion, let's say, from a bladder infection. Still, those symptoms that are likely to trouble the health worrier the most tend to be non-specific and similar from one episode to the next. They usually conjure up the thought of the same terrible disease. Often, there is a particular reason why these symptoms are frightening.

A young woman was upset by abdominal pain every week or so over a period of a half-dozen years, ever since her mother died of pancreatic cancer. She understood the connection. She was afraid that she too would get pancreatic cancer, and so she noticed pain anywhere near where she imagined the pancreas to be.

N.S.B. Case: A woman in her 30s saw a neurologist because of tension headaches that persisted day after day. She worried about a brain tumor. The following year she had somewhat different head pain from a diagnosed ear infection. Although she had all the symptoms of an ear infection, including fever and a loss of hearing, she still thought, just possibly, that she also had a brain tumor. A friend of hers had died from one.

Another N.S.B. Case: A 22 year old man who had had a single homosexual encounter seven years ago worried every time he had a skin rash that it was Kaposi's sarcoma, an incurable cancer that is also a sign of AIDS. Dermatologists assured him each time that his skin condition was benign. Each winter, the rash returned in the same areas of the body, near his ears, and went away each time with the use of a mild cortisone cream; yet each time he asked his dermatologist - the same dermatologist - whether it was possible that he might this time have Kaposi's sarcoma. Needless to say, he felt regretful and guilty about his sexual experience.

Probably the most common worry of health worriers is the fear of a heart attack. The following case history is typical:

122

A woman who was about 35 years old had a history of pressing or burning chest pain radiating into her arm. On other occasions she had shoulder pain quite distinct from the pain in her chest. Because both of her parents had died unexpectedly (in their 70s) from heart attacks, a circumstance made more vivid for her because she had witnessed their deaths, she was convinced that some day she too would die from a heart attack, even though it is a family history of prematture heart disease that is usually considered a risk factor for the disease, that is, family members dying in their 40s and 50s. Over the years her pains recurred too frequently to count. A number of different doctors performed EKGs and various other cardiac tests, all of which were reported back as normal. She was told by them that she was suffering only from tendinitis of the shoulder. Her chest pain responded to anti-inflammatory drugs. Each time the pain recurred, it faded eventually without giving any further sign of a heart attack; yet, each time she wondered if this time it was a heart attack.

Panic attacks are also very common. They affect 2 to 5% of the population with sufficient regularity as to constitute panic disorder, but occur also at a lesser frequency in a great many more people. The physical symptoms of panic disorder vary somewhat from one attack to the next, but not much. The young man described below is typical. His panic attacks started at the age of 18 and continued until he entered into cognitive-behavioral treatment at the age of 28. Among the physical symptoms he had each time were the following:

Difficulty in swallowing – which he thought might be due to a growth in his throat.

Difficulty catching his breath – which he thought might lead to choking, especially if he was eating at the time.

A light-headed feeling – which he thought might reflect an inner ear problem.

And cramps – which he thought might reflect a cancer somehow, somewhere.

Someone wearing glasses that are tinted brown tends to thinks some objects are of a brown color when they are not. If he is <u>sensible, he will recognize after a time that he is unreliable in judging</u> the color brown. He might possibly be able to judge other colors accurately even if he sees everything in a brownish direction, but his perception of brown is no good. If someone regards himself as a failure, (part of the depressive ideology) he needs to learn that his judgment of his performance will always be too pessimistic. If he wishes to see himself accurately, he must learn to compensate for that prejudice. Surely, we deal with the world more effectively if we know things the way they really are.

    <u>Similarly, if someone develops the same symptoms over and over again with no dire consequence, the next time he or she develops the same symptoms more or less, that person should understand those particular symptoms are not as serious as they seem.</u> That person is wearing glasses of a particular color. Why then do people not learn this automatically from their past experiences? The answers:

1. Because small differences are exaggerated, each experience seems different rather than similar.
2. Experiences with benign outcomes are perceived as <u>near-misses!</u> People who have panic attacks, for example, often say they <u>almost</u> choked. Or they <u>almost</u> fainted.
3. The near-misses are remembered. The far greater number of times physical symptoms come and simply go away again almost at once are forgotten.

    The solution: <u>Keep records</u>.

    Keeping records is like doing homework: no one wants to do it. Doctors do not like to keep medical records; but they do it because they have to.

    Like the other exercises suggested in this book, these records communicate a message that <u>cannot</u> be learned in any other way. For details, consult <u>Worried Sick? The Workbook</u>.

    Keep those records in as little or as much detail as you like, but every time a physical symptom appears, some record should be made. You will recognize the same symptoms appearing many times along with the same worries - each time with an uneventful recovery. If you are like most patients, you will be surprised by the great number of times the same sequence repeats. As the number of times enter into the hundreds, these records begin to make an impression. Inevitably, those particular symptoms that recur uneventfully over and over again will worry you less as time goes on.

A woman was obsessively preoccupied with breast cancer for many years for reasons that were not entirely clear to her but that had to do in part with her fear of being disfigured from radical surgery. Unfortunately, she had fibrocystic disease of the breasts, which makes them lumpy, although otherwise it is a benign condition. At her urging a surgeon had aspirated her breasts so many times she had lost count. A biopsy had been performed twice. There had never been found any indication of cancer.

Keeping records seemed to her at first to be impossible since she examined her breasts many times a day frequently finding "a new thickening or a lump." She agreed to a compromise, however, in which she kept records at least once a day. Although she thought she had understood only too well how many false alarms she had suffered through, she was still surprised to find out how often a lump she was sure was cancer disappeared a few days later. Although she always thought initially that this particular lump was a little harder or bigger than the others had been, she found she was using the same language when she was describing it for the record. Six months later, after she had begun keeping records and taking other measures such as those described below, she was able to take a different attitude summed up in her own words as: "What the hell, either I'll get cancer, or I won't." Her preoccupation with breast cancer disappeared, and she remained free of this concern for the next five years.

Everyone reacts to stress somewhat differently, and most people develop some sort of physical distress as part of that reaction.

One proctologist has said that in his experience students preparing for an examination either develop cramps and loose stools, or they become constipated. The variety of physical responses anxiety can produce is described in Chapter 12. The particular symptoms some-one experiences in the face of one kind of stress are likely to recur in similar form in the face of a different stress. Just as it is important to know the particular symptoms that concern you the most, you should know the characteristic way you react to stress; and for the same reason: in order not to confuse those symptoms with the signs of an organic illness.

It is unusual for someone who is stressed not to develop headaches or a stiff neck or low back pain or light-headedness or unsteadiness or a dry mouth or palpitations or acid indigestion or chest pain or cramps or urinary frequency or trembling or pain in the legs or arms, or <u>something</u>.

If you get stomach pains whenever your boss calls you into his office, you do not have to worry about stomach cancer the next time you get stomach pains.

If your heart starts to race whenever you have to address a meeting, you do not have to worry about an underlying cardiac disease just because your heart is beating quickly.

If you get a headache whenever you need to rush someplace – and you got a headache today rushing to pack for a trip – you do not have to worry today about a brain tumor.

On the other hand, you should see a doctor if you develop a new and persistent kind of headache. It is reasonable to see a doctor whenever you develop a new physical complaint, not necessarily because it is likely to reflect a serious condition, but because it is likely to be treatable. Sometimes the differences between an old symptom and another one only slightly different are not obvious. Record keeping helps.

<u>Know the truth about the illness you worry about.</u>

I know this is contrary to the usual medical advice. Doctors, like health worriers themselves, think that their goal should be preventing any avoidable anxiety. They are not likely to recommend that a patient read about cancer when the patient does not have cancer. They know that their patients who are health worriers react anxiously to the slightest, most peripheral, mention of their feared diseases.

A man who was afraid of having a heart attack and had gone to hospital emergency rooms 4 or 5 times with chest pain tried to avoid hearing anything about heart disease since he reacted to <u>any</u> such news with shortness of breath and a tight feeling across his chest. <u>Good</u> news about new treatments startled and distressed him seemingly as much as bad news. He gave up reading newspapers because the pages opened inevitably to the obituaries. He overheard conversations in elevators which upset him, although he was unable afterwards to repeat exactly what had been said. His doctor had taken to avoiding certain words, such as "coronary disease," to avoid frightening him; and, after his patient became upset on a few occasions encountering news about heart disease while skimming television channels, he advised him finally to stop watching television altogether! Purposely reading about heart disease would have seemed to this patient to be the height of folly. He realized, however, that his own strategy of avoidance had not worked, since every day, somehow or other, he heard about a neighbor or someone else dying suddenly from a heart attack. This is a familiar scenario to health worriers and to the people around them, especially to their doctors.

For reasons apparent in this case history, avoidance as a policy for dealing with health anxiety does not work any better than it does for any other irrational fear. The feared subject creeps in everywhere. Besides, there is no reason to be afraid. This is a man, after all, who <u>did not</u> have heart disease. The more he truly knew about heart disease, the less likely it would seem to him that he should have it. <u>Knowing a little is frightening. Knowing a lot is reassuring</u>.

When health anxiety occurs in medical students, it is often referred to as "medical student's disease." Such a medical student recognizes his own physical symptoms in the textbook descriptions of serious illness. His problem, however, is not that he knows too much; he knows too little. Even experienced physicians can know too little.

Recently, my two month old grandson skipped having a bowel movement for four days. A thought that occurred to me as a doctor was that he might have Hirshprung's disease, a condition that would not spring readily to the mind of most people. It is a rare disease that is marked by prolonged constipation and often requires surgery. I knew enough to worry, but not enough not to worry. A glance through a textbook revealed just how rare this condition is: one in 25,000 births. Also, my grandson was already past the usual age for diagnosis; and the size of his stool was not consistent with Hirshprung's disease. Also, turning the pages, I discovered that skipping a bowel movement for up to a week in infants was not uncommon and was consistent with normal development. End of worry.

2. <u>Confront your fears</u>

This could serve as a workable slogan for life itself. The fear of strangers, for instance, sets in at about 9 months of age; it is overcome by being in the company of strangers. A fear of the dark is dispelled eventually by being in the dark long enough. There is no other way. A fear of animals is managed, a little bit at a time surely, by playing with cats and dogs. A fear of performing is overcome by performing. Even the abstract fear of failure can be dispelled only by failing from time to time and learning that nothing awful follows. Every success story has featured failure along the way. Only those so determined not to fail that they never try anything fail permanently.

It is not possible to cope with an irrational fear by avoiding what is feared. Just as it is not possible to get through a week without hearing someone mention heart disease, it is not possible to live without getting sick from time to time. Facing up to getting sick and the possibility of getting very sick is part of facing up to life. Thinking the unthinkable diminishes fear. Be realistic, though. The fears health worriers can conjure up are usually worse than anything brought on by a real illness.

3. <u>Avoid checking and empty reassurance</u>.

Taking certain precautions is a proper way of dealing with danger. The caveman I referred to in a previous chapter probably posted a guard to make rounds all through the night, at least when he had spotted a saber-tooth tiger running around during the day, even when the animal turned out to be just a wild boar, or something that only looked in the distance like a saber-tooth tiger. Similarly, it makes sense for someone who lives in a bad neighborhood to make sure before going to sleep that the doors are locked. But it no longer makes sense to check the locks over and over again all through the night. Why do some people, then, check the locks, check them again a few seconds later and then again and again and again? Because the act of checking itself is comforting. No further information is obtained. No greater certainty is achieved, or safety. Unfortunately, the feeling of doubt that led in the first place to checking is unrelieved because it grows out of a sense of vulnerability that has nothing to do with any real danger. Checking makes that sense of vulnerability worse over time since it keeps the individual's attention focused on his or her fears.

There are certain precautions one can take to guard health. They are worth taking; and they should be repeated from time to time. Some of them are listed below in no special order:

1. Children should be immunized. Some of these immunizations should be repeated at intervals throughout life.

2. Children should be checked at intervals to make sure they are growing properly.

3. Certain laboratory tests should be done, probably at intervals of a few years, to pick up certain diseases of the blood, liver or kidneys that might not, if they are present, produce any overt symptoms. Diabetes can be diagnosed often by routine blood tests.

4. Throughout adulthood, blood pressure should be checked from

time to time because hypertension produces no symptoms initially and sometimes not for decades.

5. Women should check their breasts at least once a month, at most twice, to get to know how the normal breast feels. Cancers of the breast that women have picked up themselves have a better sur- vival rate than those picked up at a later date by a physician.

6. Adults should look at their skin, including their backs, every few months in order to spot early skin conditions. Some, like malig- nant melanomas, are 100% curable in early stages and 100% fatal a year later.

7. Adult women past a certain age should have PAP smears and mammograms done at intervals that may vary with age and fami- ly history. How often is still controversial.

8. Past a certain age, everyone should track cholesterol and, if it is high, the level should be lowered with diet or medication, at least in men.

9. During adulthood, rectal examination should be performed as part of a routine physical examination; and probably a chest x-ray should be taken.

10. Dental visits should be scheduled at intervals varying between 3 to 4 months and a year.

11. Later in life, colonoscopy should be performed every 8 to 10 years.

And so on.

The intervals at which these examinations should be per- formed depend on the length of time it takes for certain conditions to develop. Cervical cancer, for example, goes through a set of diag- nosable precancerous stages before it becomes invasive, and this process allows an interval of time, perhaps 2 years, during which the condition can be treated safely. Similarly, colon cancer takes a cer- tain amount of time to develop. Regular examinations at a proper interval allow sufficient time to treat polyps before they become malignant and invasive. Coronary artery disease develops over a period of many years; and it is becoming increasingly possible to intervene early in the illness in time often to prevent heart attacks or angina. Recommendations have changed over the years for the intervals between some of these examinations as more information has accumulated and a better understanding has developed about the course of these illnesses. Recently it has been suggested, for instance, that PAP smears be done less frequently and mammograms more frequently.

In short, just as making sure the front door is locked makes sense, it makes sense to check one's health in proper ways at certain times - how often depends on the particular vulnerability of the individual, which may depend in turn on many factors, including family history and the presence of certain illnesses. <u>However, it is only to a limited extent that an individual can check on his or her own health. The intervals at which that should be done should be prescribed by that person's physician. It is useless to check more frequently! Indeed, checking repetitively worsens health anxiety for the same reason checking every few seconds to see if a door is locked aggravates the concerns of an obsessive-compulsive. It focuses attention on the possibility, this next time, of finding something wrong</u>.

Health worriers not only visit doctors more frequently than they need to, or avoid them longer than they should - or both; they check their bodies much more frequently than they should. Here are some guidelines:

1. Body temperature, when you are sick, should not be checked more than once or twice a day.
2. Lumps (and lymph nodes) should not be checked for size more frequently than once a week.
3. Moles should not be checked more often than once a month.
4. Postpone to some future time checking <u>anything</u> that has remained the same the last half-dozen times you checked it.

Checking certain aspects of bodily function provides no information at all of medical significance. Do not:

1. Check the color of your urine.
2. Check the dimensions of your stool.
3. Check the coating on your tongue.
4. Check the color of your eyelids or the pouches beneath your eyes.

Another useless form of checking is to ask the same questions over and over. A doctor who thought you had a virus yesterday is likely to think so still today even if you think your condition has changed in some subtle way. Asking a spouse a medical question is obviously useless.

4. <u>Think of the odds against being desperately ill, rather than the stakes</u>

Our entire lives are governed by decisions that have a statistical quality, although we make these choices for the most part without consciously weighing the odds or even being aware that such a decision is being made. Some are more obvious than others. Some of these are precautionary. When we put on seat-belts, choose to give up smoking, drive at the speed limit, visit the dentist, put on suntan lotion, carry an umbrella, or duck when we walk through a low doorway, we are going to some trouble to avoid risk. The decision to undertake a medical treatment such as an operation is always understood explicitly in terms of risk-benefit. Sometimes because the risk is not obvious, or it is so low, we don't think of it consciously at all. When we cross an intersection with the light - or against it - we have made a decision based on an estimate of risk. The choice of whether to live in a city or in suburbia, whether or not to buy a big car, whether or not to talk back to a boss, are all made partially on the basis of an unconscious analysis of risk.

Estimating risk is a matter of knowing the odds. Most of the time-with a few striking exceptions - we know the odds well enough to get through our daily routine without notable difficulty. We learn from each other's mistakes so that most people's daily routine does not include drag-racing or eating mushrooms they have picked themselves. The exceptions are interesting. Smoking cigarettes is probably the single most dangerous activity anyone can engage in day after day. Every day smoking kills enough people to fill up a half-dozen jumbo jets. Why does a significant percentage of the population still smoke? Because most days that people smoke, they do not die! They argue from their personal, past experience; and what they read in reports of scientific studies seems remote from that day to day experience. Besides, cigarette smoking seems to them more or less under their control and is, therefore, less frightening - as opposed to panic attacks, which are, in fact, harmless, but which seem dangerous because they seem out of their control. Also, cigarettes kill people out of sight one at a time without the dramatic impact of a jumbo jet crashing at a major airport.

In some situations - airplane crashes are one -people tend to focus on the stakes rather than the odds.

"I know that mile for mile I'm safer in an airplane than traveling by car, but if the car crashes, I've still got a chance. If the plane explodes in the air, I've had it."

That person is focusing on the stakes - certain, sudden death - rather than on the odds, as he should be doing. We live-and die-by the odds. If the odds are a million to one that the plane will not crash, what difference does it make how awful a plane crash would be? Yet the stakes do matter to people. Millions of people buy lottery tickets every day dreaming about the stakes - a golden life with enough money to buy happiness, or at least a dozen expensive cars - and forgetting the odds. They see the winners on television. Nobody interviews all the losers. The odds of winning a lottery are so small that buying tickets is equivalent to throwing away money. But it is a pleasant daydream, and no one wants to think about reality.

What is harder to understand is why some people dwell so obsessively on an unpleasant daydream - illness and death - when the odds say these are very unlikely. Health worriers are concerned endlessly with the stakes - cancer, a heart attack, AIDS, a lonely and painful death in a hospital - and forget the odds. Or they do not know the odds. They argue from their daily experience - a neighbor who just had a heart attack, or today's obituaries; and they think these events are more common than they are. <u>Nobody comments on all the people who did not die yesterday or get sick today</u>. They worry for the same reason smokers do not worry: their personal experience leads them astray.

In addition, health worriers are superstitious. Among their Bad Ideas is the thought that they have been singled out for bad luck. If the chance of their having AIDS is one in a thousand, they think they will get it. Also, they think one in a hundred thousand is not much different than one in a thousand.

A number of years ago, I had an odd experience that brought home to me just how difficult it is to interpret odds. In 1981 my youngest son received 2 blood transfusions during his first attack of ulcerative colitis. A few months later the first reports of AIDS appeared in the medical literature. I was naturally concerned that he might have contracted AIDS as a result of receiving the blood. I called the local blood bank which assured me the odds were "one in a million;" but I was not comforted since at that time no one really knew what the odds were. In the next few years some statistics were reported, and I was able to figure out that the odds were actually about one in twenty-thousand. I found these really very low odds not very reassuring somehow; and on those occasions when my son got sick with anything at all, I found myself worrying about AIDS. Additional, less optimistic, statistics were reported, and I figured the odds again at, perhaps, one in a thousand. Finally, taking into consideration every unfavorable circumstance I could imagine, construing every medical report in the worst way, I figured that the odds rose to one in 200. I discovered, then, unexpectedly, that the level of my concern dropped considerably. It took me a while to understand why. The answer, I realized, was that I knew from my own experience how unlikely 1 in 200 was. All the rest were simply numbers to me. I did not ask my son to submit to an AIDS test when it became available since I knew the odds of his having the disease were exceedingly low, and I did not want to put him-and me-through the psychological difficulties attendant upon unnecessary medical testing, especially when no effective treatment was available. Now, many years later, the odds of his having contracted AIDS so long ago are about one in four million.

The trick, then, is first of all, to start thinking about the odds. If you have a swollen lymph node under your chin, what is the chance of it being due to a lymphoma compared to the chance of it being due to a sore throat? If you have a breast lump, what are the chances of it being cancer rather than a cyst? If it is a solid tumor, what are the chances of it being cancer rather than a benign fibroma? If it is cancer, what are the chances that it has already spread, rather than being still localized? If it has spread, what are the chances of it being fatal quickly rather than the kind that may kill only 20 years later? Often the incidence of a particular disease is reported in a medical textbook. Sometimes a doctor can give you a rough guess. Remember, the odds change for each condition depending on age and sex. Most illnesses are benign. Most of us get only one fatal disease per lifetime.

Second, you must recognize that the statistical laws that govern everyone else's life also rule yours. If you have been sick many times in the past, it does not mean you are more likely to get sick in the future, unless you have one of those immunological illnesses that predispose to getting sick. Third, since, like me, you may have trouble visualizing the odds, I suggest the following exercise: Mark off a thousand like this ⦀⦀ ⦀⦀ ⦀⦀ ⦀⦀ and so on until you have reached a thousand marks. It takes ten minutes. Look at the pieces of paper. You will get a feel for how unlikely it is that you will be one in a thousand. One in ten thousand is ten times less likely. You can mark that off in less than an hour and a half.

At the bottom of the page are 1500 dots. Look at the only dot printed in bold face. If you get a condition that is present in only one of fifteen hundred, that dot is you.

5. <u>Do not seek absolute certainty or safety</u>.

Some things that people do, like smoking, are so inherently dangerous that considerable effort should be exerted to avoid them. Some occupations, and certain sports, perhaps, may fall into that category, although plainly the rewards for some people outweigh the risks. Certain activities, such as gambling, or drinking alcohol, or taking illicit drugs, have such extraordinary immediate appeal that some people lose sight entirely of the risk-at least during those critical moments when temptation is strongest. Sex has this character. It is difficult to get people to engage in safe sex for long periods of time. In this matter nature has determined that we should act first and think later on. Once again, it is difficult to keep in mind scientifically proven dangers when everyday experience argues otherwise.

"I drove every day for the last month without putting on seatbelts, and nothing bad happened."

"I've been having sex for years without condoms, and I haven't caught anything yet."

In these cases, people think too much of the odds, which they misjudge, and forget the stakes altogether! But whatever the stakes, nothing in life is entirely safe.

A woman was in general very frightened. She had reached middle-age without dating much and had not traveled further than a few hundred miles from home, the same home she had lived in since she was a child. She had never married. She had few friends and was afraid of strangers. She felt unsafe trying anything new. One day she was sitting at a table in the middle of a fast-food restaurant when an automobile came through a wall - not a window - catapulted the tables nearest to the wall, and landed on her table, sending her only friend at the time to the nearest intensive care unit. Although she, herself, was uninjured, it became impossible to convince her afterwards that eating in restaurants was in general very safe.

The fact that nothing is entirely safe is not an argument for being careless. It is a reason, though, to keep in mind the law of diminishing returns, which applies to these matters as it does in every human endeavor.

A man who happened to be a physician noticed that he could palpate lymph nodes in the area of his neck, and he began to worry about developing one of those cancers, such as Hodgkin's disease, that affect lymph nodes. He was not otherwise sick. He realized that had not three of his patients recently at the same time become ill with these serious conditions, he would not have found himself examining himself for enlarged nodes. But the nodes were there. He felt them repeatedly. They were soft and not too large and not fixed to the surrounding tissues. They were probably what was left of a febrile illness he had had a month ago. Still, that was a long time for lymph nodes to linger. One node was supraclavicular, possibly a "sentinel node" which sometimes is the sign of a stomach cancer, although unlikely, the doctor thought, for a man his age without symptoms. He also wondered vaguely about lung cancer, which also seemed very unlikely since he did not smoke; but he thought to make sure by taking a chest x-ray. The x-ray was negative for cancer but was in other respects somewhat ambiguous, leading him to take skin tests for tuberculosis and sarcoidosis. The T.B. test came back equivocal, and he considered taking anti-tuberculosis drugs for a year but, on the advice of a pulmonologist who was his friend, decided instead just "to watch it." Meanwhile, he had become somewhat more worried in general. One of his patients with non-Hodgkin's sarcoma had died suddenly in an automobile accident. That this should make him more anxious about his own health seemed strange to him. At the same time one node under his chin that he had been examining every hour or so seemed to be getting larger. He decided to have it biopsied. The plastic surgeon he went to for this procedure was hesitant to perform it but went along "if it makes you feel any better." The biopsy report was lost initially but came back finally with a report "chronic non-specific inflammation." No lymphoma. For a while the doctor felt somewhat relieved, but he had now taken to

138

examining his body all over. He discovered a small lymph node in his groin which was near an unusual-looking, very subtle, skin discoloration - or so it seemed to him. Also, a lymph node near the one that had been removed began now to get larger, possibly because of a very minor wound infection at the biopsy site. A variety of other doctors were now involved. One among them suggested biopsying this new node "just to be sure."

This medical case history goes on too long to summarize briefly here. There was an additional non-diagnostic lymph node biopsy performed some time later, and other procedures. In the end most of the lymph nodes, but not all, disappeared spontaneously. The doctor never got sick.

Doctors can be health worriers, as I know from my own experience. Doctors and doctors' families tend to get more exhaustive medical work-ups than other people. This is sometimes a considerable disadvantage. Certain illnesses take a while to develop into recognizable form, and trying to rule them out prematurely is not possible. Often, as in the case described above, one is led from one obscure possibility to another. No real security can be obtained. Health anxiety is worsened by waiting for test results that can never be absolutely conclusive. Just how far to go in pursuit of an immediate diagnosis is, of course, a medical decision.

6. Live in a healthy way.

Health worriers often become preoccupied with a particular illness which may be frightening to them because they have had some incidental experience with it, such as when a family member develops the illness, or when the illness has taken on a symbolic meaning of some sort such as is often the case with sexually transmitted diseases. They may spend considerable effort warding off this illness and at the same time pay no attention to much greater dangers to their health.

A 40 year old woman was so concerned about irregularities of menstrual flow that she came when menstruating each month for the previous 15 months to some sort of emergency medical facility. She was afraid of ovarian cancer, which had affected a friend of hers. At the same time she had not visited a gynecologist for a routine check-up during the preceding ten years. She could not be persuaded to have a PAP smear, which would have picked up cervical cancer - a much more common cancer - at a treatable stage.

A middle-aged man woke up frequently with panic attacks that set his heart to beating very quickly and caused chest pain. He had gone urgently to a hospital emergency room on four occasions during the previous six months, each time convinced that he had had a heart attack. Although he was plainly terrified of dying that moment of a heart attack, which was an illusion, he showed no interest in avoiding the real, long-term dangers of heart disease! He smoked, and he routinely forgot to take medicine for the serious hypertension he had developed over a period of the last eight years.

N.S.B. Case - A woman worried about artificial dyes in food, but smoked, drank to excess and drove 80 miles per hour.

In general, it is true that health worriers are <u>less</u> likely to smoke than most people. They are also more likely to be finicky about certain foods, wary of drugs and, in general, cautious; but the exceptions are many and always surprising. As a group, they tend to exercise less than most people. They may become concerned about well-publicized, but minimal, dangers, such as radiation from power lines or lead in the drinking water, but ignore the much greater risks to health from everyday influences, especially diet.

Health worriers, like everyone else, should eat properly, exercise regularly and avoid obvious dangers, of which there are many, ranging from sunburn to falling off ladders. So much is easy to say; many others have said it. But living systematically in a healthy way is hard to do - mostly because daily habits are hard to change. Try to keep these facts in mind:

The influence of environmental factors, especially diet, on

health is tremendous. Thousands of books have been written on the proper diet. The conventional wisdom is correct: a diet with a lot of fruit and vegetables is best. At this writing, the question about whether additional vitamins should be taken is still controversial; but I believe the answer is yes. A few people for various reasons should not take extra vitamins, but the majority should. The range of illnesses that vitamins impact favorably is much greater than is generally recognized, even within the medical profession. Ideally, one's weight should be at the low part of the normal range. Do not be put off by people who say last year's dietary recommendations turn out this year to be unhealthy. There is a growing consensus about diet and health. When considering environmental risks to health, one can safely regard new dangers as greatly exaggerated and the old familiar ones as generally underestimated.

Living in a healthy way is important not only for its own sake, but because it lessens anxiety about health. Worrying is supposed to serve a purpose: it impels people to do something. The result of any effective, relevant action is to lower the level of anxiety. Exercise, in general, is better than resting.

It is readily apparent that treatment requires health worriers to behave in ways contrary to their inclinations. It is no wonder. If they were inclined naturally to confront their fears, they would not have developed health anxiety in the first place. So much is true, by the way, for all the anxiety disorders. If someone afraid of heights pushed himself to spend sufficient time looking out of tall buildings, he would soon have lost his fear of heights. If someone who got her hands dirty did not wash at the first opportunity, she would not have developed the sense of contamination that underlies a hand-washing compulsion. Reversing these habits of avoidance is not easy.

The six principles mentioned above have to be embodied in a specific program of treatment (See Worried Sick? The Workbook). It is helpful, of course, for the health worrier to keep in mind the facts described in previous chapters about the nature of physical illness, the ways doctors think, and so on; but the fixed attitudes with which health worriers come to treatment are difficult to change by what amounts to a formal lecture. Their previous experience of life, colored by distortions of perception and memory, argue otherwise. Real cure comes from experiencing the world anew. Certain behavioral exercises, engaged in systematically, have been found to be effective. Thought, feeling and behavior are inextricably intertwined and changing one changes the others. The influence of one on the other may seem paradoxical at first glance. Consider a woman who is afraid of germs and washes her hands compulsively. One might think naively that proper treatment would mean convincing that woman somehow that germs are not dangerous to her, after which she would spontaneously stop washing. It turns out the most effective treatment requires the patient to stop washing - after which the thought of germs and the attendant feeling of contamination disappears!

A number of clinical strategies can be undertaken to implement the six principles. None of them are congenial to the health worrier. They are reported in the next chapters.

Chapter Eight: Seven Ways to Break the Pattern

The principles by which people live have to be reduced to specific ways of behaving in order for those principles to have meaning. It is one thing, for instance, to profess love for one's neighbor as one loves oneself, but the meaning invested in that idea comes from the way someone behaves across a backyard fence. Learning new ways of thinking is like learning a new skill; it requires some effort and practice. It cannot be accomplished just by reading a book of directions. Learning to swim implies getting in the water. Knowing theoretically that human beings can float is no help. So, this is an argument for actually doing those specific cognitive-behavioral exercises which in our program and in others have been found to be helpful in treating health anxiety - and not doing other things which make health anxiety worse.

1. Research the Disease You Fear.

The natural inclination of health worriers is to avoid hearing or reading anything about disease in general and in particular about whichever disease haunts them the most. When they cannot turn away, literally, it is not uncommon for them to hold their hands over their ears, as if the words themselves - cancer, heart attack - have the capacity to injure! Certainly, these words are painful. Hearing unexpectedly that a neighbor has cancer causes a shock that has a distinctly physical aspect to it, like an electric shock. Often it is not possible to communicate good news to health worriers because using these words in a sentence causes them to fidget and look about nervously. They are distracted by an emotionally charged image so subtle it is largely unconscious. The words become the thing itself. The identification with the sick neighbor is so immediate and powerful, it is as if for just a moment they themselves had the cancer. Like a rat that has been conditioned to avoid an electric shock, health worriers become averse to hearing mere words. But cancer and heart disease and other various afflictions are in the news all the time; and so these men and women are continually disturbed anew. Health worriers must be desensitized to the language of disease before they can find out enough about a particular illness to recognize that they are safe.

There are a number of emotional disorders that are similar to health anxiety in that they are based on an irrational fear. Some of these, such as phobias or obsessive-compulsive disorder, have been described briefly. The fears that drive them are obvious; but there are others, such as the sexual dysfunctions, where the underlying fears are more obscure. The cognitive behavioral treatments for all these various disorders have certain elements in common.

A. The feared object or situation must be approached purposely and systematically rather than having it thrust upon the patient inadvertently or unexpectedly. It is important for the patient to feel in control.

B. Confronting the feared object or situation should be accomplished a little bit at a time. Sometimes the presence of someone who is unafraid is helpful since a sense of calm is contagious just as in a different context a frightened feeling may be contagious.

C. Long periods of exposure work better than multiple short exposures. It is important for the patient to have time to calm down while still in the frightening situation.

It is a good idea for you to follow this model while researching the illness you worry about. First of all: make up your mind not to turn off the television set, fold the newspaper, or walk away from the person talking to you when the subject comes up. Read more. Draw the person out. Try to cultivate a perverse sense of satisfaction from doing the right thing, even when that thing is uncomfortable. It is akin to the gratification a fatigued athlete gets after a difficult workout. Get the morbid details. Will you feel anxious? Certainly. Consider the discomfort an investment in the future. Just as someone afraid of the water finds learning to swim an uneasy process, so will you have to pay a price to overcome your fears.

Pursuing the subject rather than avoiding it, you will discover

144

to your surprise, if you keep track of such things, that the facts of the matter you are hearing about may not be as you imagined. The neighbor who had cancer did not have cancer after all. She was only tested for cancer. Or she had a cancer that the doctors caught in time. Or she had a cancer that resulted from exposure to a chemical that you have never been near during the course of your life. Sometimes the news account is not of someone dying prematurely from a heart attack, but of a new drug or vitamin treatment. Folic acid, most recently, has been found to reduce the chance of a heart attack. You will also start running into a number of people who have had heart attacks, or cancer, or whatever, and nevertheless continue to live decently, without worrying constantly about the immanence of death. Sometimes, when such a person has a devastating illness, his or her life is described by others as inspiring. And it is. But I think that managing to live on in such a way is more the rule than the exception.

Then, secondly, go out of your way to read articles in the popular press, or anywhere else, on the subject of the disease you fear. However, do not take what you read seriously. These accounts are selective and, as everyone knows, distorted by the various reportorial and editorial changes that take place between the time of the interview with the doctor and the time the report of the interview reaches print. Putting it bluntly, what appears in the lay press is often wrong. As a physician, I have trouble reconstructing from reading a magazine article what the doctor who was the source of the information must have intended to say. When I read in a magazine what I myself was supposed to have said in an interview, I often cannot make sense of it. Sometimes the reporter makes me sound sensible. Sometimes I sound like an idiot. But I never sound like myself. But not all the information appearing in the popular press is wrong. Even if only a little is learned, that much is useful. Indeed, the value of this exercise is primarily in exposing yourself purposely to a frightening idea. Inevitably, with systematic exposure, your level of anxiety will drop.

Finally, however, it becomes important to know the truth about the feared illness. The truth is not easy to learn, even for someone who is not trying to run away. There are a few, if not many, good books written for lay people on the most serious illnesses; and I recommend starting with them. The only other reliable sources of information are the internet, medical text books and your physician. Your physician, if he is like most, will have little patience for your interrogating him about a disease you do not have, so he must be used for this purpose rarely and as a last resort only to clear up lingering questions.

I have misgivings recommending to patients that they read a medical textbook. For one thing, such advice is followed rarely. Besides, these texts are not easily available, and they are not easy to read. The terminology cannot be readily understood by someone who is not trained medically. After all, they are intended for medical students and for doctors. Worse, they emphasize all the complications of the disease even when such problems are quite rare. They give worst-case scenarios. Still, what health worriers need to know is obtainable most readily in medical textbooks, that is:

1. Who gets the disease?

The peculiar problem I had all my life with my memory (trouble with names and numbers) seemed to get worse in medical school. I wondered if I could be suffering an early-onset presenile dementia. Opening a textbook at the right page revealed that early-onset dementia always starts much later in life.

A young man was afraid he had stomach cancer. I was able to take down a medical textbook and show that he too was the wrong age for the disease he was worrying about.

A woman thought she might (with her luck) give birth to a Tay Sachs baby as a friend of hers just did. Wrong background. Tay Sachs disease, a devastating illness that causes rapid physical deterioration and death in the first few years of life, occurs primarily in Jews of European extraction.

146

Another woman, who had muscle cramps, was afraid that she had muscular dystrophy. Wrong sex. At her age only men get muscular dystrophy.

Many, if not most, diseases occur preferentially in one sex, or at a certain age, or in men and women of one or another ethnic background or race. Often, the disease is relatively rare in the first place. Textbooks report the incidence and prevalence of all the medical illnesses. Some, such as the tropical diseases, occur only in certain countries and certain climates.

2. How does the disease present?

Each illness has a characteristic course. It starts in a certain way, develops a pattern after a time by which it becomes recognizable, and has one of a limited number of outcomes.

A young man with a family history of colon cancer got cramping pain in the lower side of the abdomen whenever he got upset. When he did not think he might have an acute appendicitis, he was worried that he might have colon cancer. But colon cancer, he was told by his gastroenterologist, does not start with pain. It starts with bleeding and anemia. He was the wrong age too.

A young woman regularly developed chest pain after meals. She worried about heart attacks. But heart attack pain is not relieved, as hers was, by antacids. And considering her age, she was the wrong sex.

A man with chronic frontal headaches and swelling below his eyes worried about having a brain tumor. But he ran a fever along with the headaches, and fever is not a symptom of brain tumors. He had a sinusitis.

Another man, who had panic attacks, was afraid he might be developing Grand Mal epilepsy. He had once seen someone having an epileptic attack in the street. But Grand Mal epilepsy causes a loss of consciousness, which had never happened to him.

Health anxiety is an exaggerated and, consequently, unwarranted fear of illness. It follows then, obviously, that the more health worriers know about such an illness, the more discrepancies will become apparent between the symptoms of that condition and their own symptoms. It is particularly important to note the order in which symptoms develop.

If someone develops breast pain from cancer, it is only after other symptoms have appeared; namely, a mass.

Someone does not develop swollen legs from heart failure without a history of heart disease and a half-dozen other symptoms.

Pain is not the first sign of a stroke.

And so on.

I grant there are exceptions to the usual course of a disease often enough to make the practice of medicine challenging and not something that can be done simply by leafing through a textbook and checking off the appropriate box. There are patterns to the exceptions also, and sometimes exceptions to those exceptions. Nevertheless, health worriers do not have to be medically knowledgeable to recognize that they should not think of a particular deadly disease when they do not have the symptoms of that condition, especially if their symptoms are consistent with a much more common condition.

Remember, think horses, not zebras.

In addition to reading about feared diseases, health worriers should try to find out as much as possible about those illnesses that they <u>do</u> have. The more they know, the less likely are they to worry about the wrong condition. Certain illnesses are routinely confused by healthy worriers and they are discussed in greater length in Chapter 11.

These are:

Gastro-esophageal reflux disorder (GERD), vs. heart disease.

Muscular-skeletal disease (chest wall) vs. heart attack.

Vascular and/or tension headaches vs. brain tumor.

Irritable bowel syndrome vs. colon cancer.

Sometimes a panic disorder is confused with going crazy. This last category contrasts two purely emotional diseases and is worth considering separately for this reason.

Panic Attacks vs. Going crazy

Health worriers often include mental disease among their pre-occupations. They ask if those strange feelings they have been having recently are an indication of schizophrenia or some other psychosis. Often these feelings are what are called "panic attacks." It is a very common condition affecting, perhaps, 5% or more of the population. A typical panic attack has both a physical and a psychological dimension.

Physically: suddenly the individual notices palpitations, light-headedness, a sense of imbalance, trouble catching his or her breath or difficulty swallowing, pain in the chest and weakness or shaking in any of the limbs.

Psychologically: There is the fear of fainting or screaming or acting in some embarrassing or dangerous manner, such as driving a car off a bridge or into a crowd. These are behaviors someone may ordinarily associate with being crazy. In reality, no such loss of control occurs in a panic attack. There is no report of any person having had an automobile accident in the midst of such an attack. The only truly embarrassing behavior panicky persons engage in frequently is to leave peremptorily whatever social situation they may be in when they become panicky. Someone who customarily avoids or withdraws from such a place is said to be phobic for that place. Someone who avoids many places because of the fear of being trapped there with a panicky feeling is usually called agoraphobic.

Panic disorder is a good example of a condition that produces striking and complicated physical symptoms which have, however, no clinical significance. In fact, cure comes finally only when the individual becomes blasé about becoming panicky; and strange as it seems to speak in such terms, that is the usual result of proper treatment. Schizophrenia, on the other hand, and the other psychotic states which seem to the health worrier to underlie the panic attack, are an entirely different matter. They have their own causes and their own symptoms. Schizophrenia, for example, is manifest in peculiar disturbances of thought and feeling, difficult to describe briefly. As often as not, a psychotic episode begins with a paranoid state characterized by hallucinations and delusions. In contrast to the panicky person, it does not often occur to a psychotic that he might in fact be crazy.

In each of the illnesses mentioned above, and in all others, knowing the exact shape of the condition is, in the end, reassuring because it allows the health worrier to distinguish his or her symptoms from those that characterize the fearful illness he or she has in mind.

2. Dwell on your "nightmare" fantasy purposely!

All emotional states fade. Grief lasts normally only a number of months. Sadness, fear, lust, rage: these all fade with time unless some new circumstance causes them to flare into existence again. Even those who know - who do not simply imagine - that they have cancer, come to a period of time when they think of it only occasionally and occupy themselves instead with their usual concerns, which may have to do with work or family or those idiosyncratic preoccupations that make each one of us the particular person we are. In a way we are all living under a death sentence, for we will all die some day. The person who knows he will probably die of his cancer some day does not know that date any more than the rest of us know the date we will die. It seems to most of us, most of the time, that today will not be that day. Emotions are a signal to act, and when effective action is not possible, the emotion dies away. Fear fades away with time. We can help the process along.

Most of us remember an occasion when we mulled over endlessly some embarrassing incident or failure. At first the memory rankles, but then becomes less upsetting as time goes on. Finally, we can remember the incident without distress. Similarly, someone abandoned by a lover will be saddened going to a place the two of them had previously frequented together, but less and less sad as time goes on, after revisiting that place again and again. All memories lose their emotional accent over time. They become matter-of-fact. It is only when the thought of a particular experience is avoided that it returns painfully against our wishes. Such is the character of the emotional problems that occur subsequent to a traumatic event. In that situation symptoms grow out of the wish not to remember. A thought that is intentionally put out of mind, whether it is of an automobile accident or the possibility of developing cancer will erupt at a later time unpredictably and often over and over again. People say that time heals; but it is not time per se, but the re-experiencing of events in a non-threatening setting. This process is called desensitization; and to some extent it can be accomplished in the mind. Just as someone can become blasé at the thought of becoming panicky, someone can learn to contemplate death itself with equanimity. There is a report in the medical literature of someone who overcame his fear of fatal illness in as little as a week by concentrating on and imagining the process of dying. For an hour a day. The fear of death is not always what it seems to be though; and the process of overcoming it is usually more complicated than this last example would suggest.

A patient in our health anxiety clinic who happened to be a physician said that his awful imaginings were of being told by his doctor: "Sit down, please. I'm afraid I have some bad news for you. The laboratory report on your biopsy has come back, and you were right. It's non-Hodgkin's lymphoma." In this fantasy the doctor then goes on patiently, sympathetically, to remark on the optimistic aspects of the case; but, of course, the truth, known to our patient, is that there is no reliably successful treatment, and the condition is likely to be fatal in a short period of time. It is this scene that loomed in the mind of the health worrier.

This is about as far - even further - than most nightmare fantasies go. It is often a single picture, or a bit of dialogue, from which the health worrier withdraws with a shudder. It is a bit of awfulness "What if..." that frightens in and of itself. There is no consideration given to afterwards. There is no examining of the scene for the real likelihood of it ever taking place. It is as much a feeling as a thought.

So, the patient was told to think that terrifying thought and feel that feeling as deeply as he could, purposely, for an hour a day - from 5 o'clock in the afternoon to 6 o'clock. He was asked also to postpone his worrying until that time. Of course, this is not easy to do. The thought and feeling rose up as usual in his mind 30 or 40 times a day when for no obvious reason he remembered the somewhat enlarged lymph node that was the current reason for his worrying. Somehow, however, with practice, with the real distractions of real life, and with the knowledge that later on he would be worrying, he was able to get through most mornings and afternoons more comfortably than usual. But neither was it easy for him to dwell on his nightmare fantasy for a whole hour every day, not because it seemed perverse-which it did - and not because it was agonizing - for it was not - but because after 10 or 15 minutes, it was boring. In order to muster up the dismay he usually felt pondering this imaginary scene he had to elaborate on the details. Perhaps his doctor told him also that the disease had already spread. Maybe his wife was in the room; and she had begun crying. Maybe he imagined himself fainting after hearing the bad news.

In the ensuing weeks these first scenes he imagined seem to lose their impact; but others could be conjured up that could elicit that same awful feeling. He imagined himself alone in a hospital bed, wasting away, being fed intravenously, calling for the nurse at night with no one to answer. Finally, he imagined himself dead from the cancer. He lay in the casket knowing he had had no time to have children or practice his profession. He imagined himself being alone forever.

It took weeks of practice to think of these desperate scenes without getting upset; but that time came.

It seems the fear of dying is really in most cases the fear of being helpless, usually in the indifferent hands of doctors and nurses, or the fear of being alone. Sometimes, however, it is a different thing, such as the fear of becoming physically ugly, which is the way some people see the process of dying. Breast cancer may be threatening because it implies disfigurement and the loss of sexual identity. It is hard to put a good face on developing a fatal illness and dying, but having seen many people die, I have to say that it is not as bad as most health worriers imagine. In this respect, as in so many others, their fears are unrealistic. Most people are still in control of their lives-as much as they ever were-and most people die more or less in the company of their families. Often they are too sleepy to care if someone is sitting with them or not. The average hospital death is not terribly painful, more uncomfortable. I would just as soon skip the whole business myself, but given the alternative of dying suddenly in my sleep or slowly over the course of a week with time to say goodbye to the people I care about, I would prefer the latter. So:

1. Try to define exactly what it is you imagine when you imagine yourself seriously ill.
2. Dwell on that possibility as if it were real for an hour a day, meanwhile trying to put that fear out of mind the rest of the time.
3. If you cannot feel that awful sense of dread throughout the entire hour-if you find your mind wandering-try changing the daydream into something worse: physical pain, increasing enfeeblement, family distress, depression, death itself, perhaps even the entombment that comes after death.

The exact shape of the nightmare that comes to mind finally, may be surprising and often illuminates the otherwise unconscious concerns that drive the health anxiety.

Another patient in the same health anxiety clinic, a woman, found herself haunted by a particular image: <u>What if</u> she had a heart attack while walking through a department store with her 5 year old daughter? <u>What if</u>, then, someone kidnapped her child?

I leave it to the reader to, work out the psychological dynamics implicit in such a narrative. In order truly to understand that meaning, though, one would have to know that particular person. Also, conversely, knowing that person would be easier if one keeps in mind those fears expressed so clearly in her nightmare fantasy. It would be wonderful if it were possible in such a way to really understand patients, or anyone at all, for that matter, in the profound way psychoanalysis seemed to promise 50 or 60 years ago. The bad news is that it is not possible. The good news is that it is not necessary in order to relieve those emotional problems with which this book deals.

At first glance it would seem that many people share the same health worries; but as every person is unique so are their ideas about illness and of death.

Two men came to see me, one within a number of months of the other, both complaining of a fear of having contracted AIDS. AIDS is a common concern among those who are preoccupied with their health, first, of course, because it is fatal and second, because some can harbor the virus with very little or no obvious physical symptoms. As is normally the case with such patients, neither had but the most far-fetched reasons for thinking he might have been exposed to the virus. As a matter of fact, both had tested negatively within the previous few months but continued worrying nevertheless. After all, the test is not always accurate. When encouraged to make explicit their nightmare fantasies, though, he were very different. One man pictured himself shriveled and weak and shunned by everyone. It was a scenario of humiliation and of having become abhorrent to everyone. The second man saw himself tied to a hospital bed by tubes of all sorts. He pictured himself too weak to move.

He was by himself, listening to other people playing ball outside his hospital window. His fantasy was of being helpless and alone.

Both men had lived lives which were consistent with their individual concerns even prior to their having heard about AIDS. The first man was a weight-lifter who had always felt he was too thin. The second man was the youngest of four siblings and had always felt left out by his family.

You must desensitize yourself to your own particular nightmare fantasy.

However it is important to keep reality in mind even when fantasizing. Even as you imagine some terrible, worst-case scenario, remind yourself of the odds against this fantasy ever coming true. And think the fantasy through to the end. After all, the diagnosis of cancer, for instance, is by no means a death sentence. <u>What if...</u> is often followed by a reasonable <u>well, then...</u>

Some examples:

"<u>What if</u> this lump in my breast is not a cyst like last time, but a tumor?"

"<u>Well, then</u>, the tumor can be removed. Many breast tumors are benign."

"But <u>what if</u> the tumor is malignant?"

"<u>Well, then</u>, there is still a good likelihood that you caught it in time, especially since you have been going for routine mammograms and regular check-ups."

"<u>What if</u> the cancer has spread nevertheless?"

"<u>Well, then</u>, there is still a good chance that surgery plus chemotherapy and radiation will destroy the cancer or prevent its return."

"<u>What if</u> the cancer doesn't respond to those treatments?"

"<u>Well, then</u>, breast cancer spreads, sometimes, so slowly it may not shorten your life span."

And so on.

"<u>What if</u> this chest pain turns out to be a heart attack?"

"Well, then, you go to an emergency room. There are new treatments that can dissolve the clot if you get there within a few hours."

"But what if I can't get there in time?"

"Well, then, you will need to undertake a program of rehabilitation and probably have to take medication. Most first heart attacks do not prove to be fatal."

"What if I have to stop working because of my heart attack?"

"Well, then, you may be able to do other kinds of work. Or you can live off your disability insurance."

"But, what if...

"What if my condition gets worse on vacation?" "Well, then, you can call one of the local doctors." "What if there is no doctor on that island?" "Well, then, you can bring along extra medicine." "What if the medicine gets lost along with my other baggage?' "Well, then, you can take the ferry that leaves the island to go to the mainland every afternoon." "What if there is a storm and the ferry can't put to sea?"

Etc.

But keep in mind the odds.

What are the chances that the lump in your breast is really cancer when it was a cyst the last time?

What are the chances that the cancer is inoperable when it is of recent onset?

What are the chances that your chest pain is a heart attack when each time over the last 10 years it turned out to have a different cause?

What are the chances of an island with 50,000 residents not having a doctor?

I know it is hard to believe that a mental exercise intended to make you feel bad will make you better in the long run, but in other guises this strategy of confrontation seems more familiar.

156

In order to overcome a fear of public speaking, one has to- a little bit at a time, perhaps-get up in front of groups and speak, which will surely make anyone anxious the first dozen or so times.

A fear of contamination is overcome by purposely soiling one's hands and refraining from washing. This is exceedingly unpleasant for the first 10 or 20 hours!

A fear of a boss can be eliminated only by talking to him. Some bosses assume mythic proportions if they can get away with it. Talking with him the first few times may seem threatening, and will be upsetting, but not after a while.

All of these situations are threatening at first only because they suggest a danger which turns out later on to be illusory. In the absence of a real illness the only way the dangers of being sick can be confronted is by thinking them through systematically. (See chapter 9 for a more detailed examination of nightmare fantasies.)

3. Exercise!

Health worriers have certain Bad Ideas about their bodies. Often they feel they are:

A. Too fat or too skinny.

B. Weak.

C. Too easily tired, too vulnerable to infection, too subject to drug reactions, too allergic, too sensitive to stress. And for all these reasons,

D. Sickly.

The reasons why they have grown up believing themselves to be fragile and sickly have been described previously. Can anything be done now, years later, to change those attitudes? Sure. But not without difficulty.

It is easy to see that someone capable of running a marathon is not likely to overreact to shortness of breath or to his heart beating quickly. That person experiences those particular physiological changes throughout the race, along with sweating, light-headedness, thirst and various physical pains. That person is accustomed to these physical responses and regards them as normal. If someone who worries about such "symptoms" can be persuaded to become a long-distance runner, these preoccupations inevitably disappear. Nor is someone capable of running hours on end likely to regard himself or herself as infirm, whatever that person may have felt growing up. So, I recommend to my readers that they become long-distance runners. You are not planning to take that advice? I am not surprised. What is surprising is that a few patients have indeed become marathoners. Their concerns about their physical health have disappeared along the way.

Running a marathon may be out of the reach of most people, but regular exercise is possible for everyone. There are health benefits to exercise over and above the psychological benefits. Coronary artery disease, diabetes, hypertension, cardiac arrhythmias, osteoporosis and perhaps a dozen other physical illnesses are either prevented or ameliorated by regular exercise. Those who have been seriously ill recently, let's say from a heart attack, are usually encouraged to enter into a supervised program of exercise as soon as possible. Health worriers are often troubled by chronic diseases that are real and troublesome; and they may, then, be forced to exercise less vigorously than they would be capable of doing otherwise; but within the limitations of proper medical advice, everyone should exercise. Longevity is correlated unmistakably with fitness.

Whether you have been recently ill, or not; whether you have been diagnosed with "chronic fatigue syndrome" or some other more or less debilitating condition, you can exercise to some extent and in time become relatively fit. And it feels good. Try to imagine being able to walk more briskly than the people around you, running up a flight of stairs instead of walking, feeling energetic instead of being tired all the time, looking younger in the mirror. These pleasures come with exercise, along with the more subtle satisfaction of engaging successfully in a difficult task. Exercise itself becomes pleasurable after the first month or so, so much that some people are said to be "addicted" to exercising. Certainly there are people who go jogging, for example, in all kinds of weather. There is some reason to think that - for some people at least - exercising may have an anti-depressant effect. Some people report that they worry less after jogging than they did before setting out.

I know this advice is no more congenial than my other recommendations. Health worriers are precisely that group of people who feel too tired, too sick or just too worn out to exercise today. Maybe tomorrow, but not today. If they were more inclined to exercise, they would likely not have this problem in the first place. Feeling less strong than other people, they feel less capable of exercising. They rest a lot. Consequently, they become weaker. This sense of physical incapacity can become extreme. The treatment is exercise!

How much exercise is desirable? The answer depends on a number of factors, including age and health. A doctor's advice may be desirable. For most people, however, I think 4 to 7 hours a week is optimum. This may seem like a lot, but my purpose is to encourage health worriers to think that they are capable of a lot. As they are.

How should you start? Assuming that you think that exercising vigorously is probably desirable, but way too hard for you, start small. Assuming you have been told a hundred times before to exercise, but have not gotten around to it, start very small. You do not have to get into shape today. Begin today. It is better to begin with an hour of very light exercise than with 10 minutes of vigorous exercise. There is no reason to make this business any more unpleasant than necessary. In fact, you have an <u>obligation</u> to make it as easy as possible since otherwise you will surely give up. Being physically active is inherently pleasurable, but not at first. If you can keep going for only a matter of weeks by an effort of will, you will keep going afterwards because you will want to exercise for its own sake.

<u>Four Things not to do.</u>
1. Do not check your symptoms over and over again.

Somebody about to set off on a trip to another country checks every few minutes to see if he still has his passport and airline tickets. Before leaving, his wife checks the back door twice to make sure it is locked. Both of them check the time of their flight repeatedly to make sure they don't arrive late.

Probably this vignette sounds familiar. Confronting a critical event, most people become anxious and engage in checking behavior to make sure their plans are not going awry. This is not entirely irrational. At some time or other everyone has forgotten to set an alarm or bring along an appointment book. Everyone at one time or another has omitted doing something important only to catch the error at the last minute by checking. Sometimes, however, these defensive maneuvers become exaggerated and then take on a life of their own. In order to ward off danger, a person may make her way around her house every evening checking to see if the windows and doors are locked and the gas stove is turned off and then, never entirely certain she was careful enough, do it a second time, and then a third, fourth and fifth time. Probably any psychological defense can be taken to an extreme and become pathological and perverse. Someone inclined to avoid conflict can become reclusive. Someone else can carry being assertive to the extent of becoming truculent. Someone suspicious of the motives of others can verge into being overtly paranoid. And so on. The person who checks endlessly is said to be obsessive-compulsive. Such a person may also have fears of germs and contamination, which may be warded off by washing rituals, the essence of which is once again constant repetition. In some individuals there is an overlap between obsessive-compulsive disorder and health anxiety.

A woman noticed at the age of 45 a bump at the back of her skull at about the level of her ears. Despite being told by her doctors that these were lymph nodes and had no clinical significance, she palpated them a half-dozen times a day over a period of weeks to see if they were growing. Ultimately they began to hurt her, solely because she was examining them so vigorously.

A man with a lingering viral disease and a low-grade fever checked his temperature 7 or 8 times each evening although the level of his fever did not vary by more than a half-degree from one day to the next over a period of weeks.

N.S.B. Cases:

An elderly woman checked each morning of the last 20 years to see if her tongue was coated. She may in the distant past have had a yeast infection in her mouth, but she had been free of all symptoms and certainly free of any clinically diagnosable mouth disorder ever since.

A balding young man counted the hairs in the sink each time he washed his hair. Seeing them lying there caused him "angst." (His word.) It means, according to Webster's 3rd unabridged dictionary: a feeling of anxiety: dread, anguish. His distress was so great he refrained from washing his hair for weeks at a time. Consequently, he developed an unsightly scalp seborrhea, something like cradle cap in babies. This condition may have accelerated his hair loss.

An adolescent boy who was worried that drugs he was taking for an inflammatory condition were stunting his growth checked his height 3 or 4 times a day over a period of months. He was surprised to note that his height varied over the course of each day by over one-half inch. Month by month, however, he grew normally. During adolescence, health anxiety seems to merge with concerns about appearance, and it is not uncommon for kids to stare into a mirror seemingly all day long to check their acne or whether or not their breasts are growing symmetrically.

There are reports in the medical literature of individuals who have examined parts of their bodies so vigorously and constantly that these organs have become inflamed and required surgical removal. These have included a salivary gland in one person and a testicle in another. I have seen a woman who caused an abscess to form in a breast by examining it persistently for lumps.

Almost any aspect of bodily functioning can be checked compulsively by health worriers. Many people check their pulse throughout the day, sometimes so frequently that one hand is kept unconsciously on the other wrist even when not measuring the pulse. Others check blood pressure, or menstrual flow, or the character of their bowels or their urine. Checking to see if one's balance is slightly askew will cause a defect in balance. Some people count their breaths. Many times attention is given to a part of the body which does not commonly reflect any disease. For example, one woman worried whether the veins of her hands were becoming more prominent; and she would stare at them from time to time.

What is happening psychologically to drive this behavior, which seems on the face of it to accomplish nothing? The affected individuals report simply that they are worried and are seeking only to make sure they have no reason to worry. But why do they check again and again? Because, they reply, they are not completely, absolutely, entirely sure they checked properly. They do not remember hearing the click of the door when they tried to lock it. Was the knob on the gas range really turned all the way counter-clockwise, or was it off by a few degrees? When they were washing, did the dirty part of their hand touch the clean part, making the clean part dirty? It is as if compulsive individuals do not trust their senses-or, at least, the memory of what their senses tell them. One treatment technique that has proven helpful to such patients is to get them to slow down their compulsive rituals. They turn off the stove so slowly and exactly, they experience the act differently. Changing compulsive behavior in any way at all is often helpful.

Those who check their bodies compulsively are doing something similar. They too forget whether their pulse was 84 a minute ago or, just possibly, 86. And they don't remember exactly the feel of the lump. But even if they did remember, that was then and this is now. They are monitoring their physical condition to see if it changes. What is extraordinary is that they are under the impression that they are checking in order to reassure themselves, yet the inevitable outcome of that persistent examination is to leave them still uncertain and anxious. For one thing, they share a mistaken idea that very slight variations - in heart rate, for example, or body temperature - are clinically significant. In fact, the act of checking itself can cause variations in function - heart rate is an example again, or blood pressure - which they may interpret as abnormal.

The real reasons why people check can be better understood by examining the emotional context in which they engage in these behaviors rather than by simply asking them for their reasons. They start off suspecting that they may be seriously ill. They may feel bad physically, and feel anxious and depressed about feeling bad. In the face of what seems like an immediate danger, they examine themselves warily with the vague idea that they may discern the enemy from a far enough distance to be able to take counter-measures in time. If the doctors are the generals, they are the scouts. At that moment there is some diminution of anxiety, first, because action of any sort tends to diminish the level of emotional arousal – and, secondly, because most of the time the enemy has not appeared or if he is in sight, he has not come any closer. The lump is no bigger than it was a few minutes ago. The fever is no worse. There is a momentary sense of relief. But the underlying presumption that they are ill has not gone away and begins to assert itself again more strongly the more time passes. Checkers do not remember well the results of their last examination. Ambiguity creeps in. The urge builds to do again something that is at least in some small way comforting. And they check again. Less apparent to them is the fact that the act of checking itself keeps in sharp focus the possibility of their getting sick or sicker. The danger looms before them continuously; and their fear grows. In short, they check <u>not because checking provides any new information or relevant information</u>, but because it causes their anxiety level to drop momentarily. At the cost of making them worry more and more.

So, don't check.

There are, of course, times when it is appropriate to examine one's body. Examples have been given in a previous chapter. Health worriers do better, though, by erring on the side of not checking. These are reasonable rules to follow:

a. Follow your doctor's advice. If she advises you to keep track of your temperature or examine a mole to see if it is getting larger, or check your breasts for lumps, do so; but do so only as frequently as she advises, no more, no less. If she suggests you keep track of some symptom, but neglects to tell you how often you should check, ask her to be specific.

b. Do not examine your body in ways which you know ahead of time will give you no meaningful information. For example, do not bother to determine if your veins are becoming more prominent, or if your tongue is coated. Also, do not press on a part of your body to see if doing so causes more pain that the last time you pressed on it. Do not work your joints to see if they make noise. Do not monitor your appetite so that you can see if you really get hungry when you think you should be getting hungry. Do not worry if your urine is too yellow, or not yellow enough. The body functions differently under different circumstances; and not every variation from the usual pattern is an indication of illness. If you are inclined to check some aspect of your body's functioning on the assumption that that aspect of function is meaningful to health, check first with your physician.

    If you think you are slowly falling apart by virtue of growing old, do not monitor the deterioration carefully. There is no point in checking to see just how grey, bald, wrinkled or slow-witted you are becoming. These are not signs of disease in the conventional sense.

c. Keep in mind that there is a range through which certain aspects of bodily function can vary normally, so that knowing whether you fall this minute at one extreme or the other, or someplace in between, is not helpful in determining how healthy you are. Blood pressure, for instance, can be, and should be, elevated during physical exercise or emotional excitement. It can drop quite low normally if someone is dehydrated or has just taken a hot bath. In diagnosing essential hypertension, it is important to know how high the pressure goes <u>when the individual is relaxed</u>. How high it goes when the patient is upset-perhaps simply by having his blood pressure taken- is less significant. Health worriers often run a higher blood pressure at the beginning of a physical examination than a half-hour later. Similarly, the rate of breathing, heart beat, and frequency of urination varies within wide limits normally. Some people become greatly worried if they move their bowels somewhat less frequently than usual. I found a report in the medical literature of a man who moved his bowels once every six months.[1]

If you are truly ill, the parameters of that illness may vary over the course of a day or so without giving any indication about whether that condition is improving or worsening. Most fevers, for example, go down in the mornings and up in the evenings no matter how sick the person is. Cardiac arrhythmias may be a little more or less obvious at different times during a day for no important reason. The pain of a gall-bladder attack may depend on what you eat and is not an accurate guide to determining whether the condition is getting better or worse. Breast lumps may change in size relative to different times in a menstrual cycle without indicating any change in the underlying condition. These are all reasons for not bothering to keep very close tabs on physical symptoms. They do not always reflect the course of the illness that causes them. Physical symptoms that change consistently over time in a particular direction are more like-

---

[1] I assume that there is someone else someplace who moves his bowels only once a year but has not gotten around to talking to his doctor about it. On the other hand, as an intern I was awakened one morning at 3 A.M. by a man who called urgently to complain that he had not been able to move his bowels since midnight.

ly to be significant. Subtle changes are not likely to have clinical significance.

d. Do not bother to check any element of physical health, or any physical symptom, that has not changed during the last half-dozen times you checked it. Presumably, the only rational reason for paying attention to physical symptoms is to be in position to take action quickly should an illness suddenly become evident or worsen critically. Most illnesses, however, can be treated just as effectively tomorrow as today. No physical illness mild enough to be managed at home needs to be monitored closely hour by hour or minute by minute. The very minimal benefit of beginning a new treatment early is outweighed by the psychological disadvantages of frequent checking, which probably has physical ill-effects, also, through the mechanisms of stress. Besides, as a watched pot never boils, physical symptoms you check on every minute never go away.

I think most health worriers come to understand that their checking does no good but they find it harder to believe that it actively worsens their fears. But it does.

A patient, who happened be a psychiatrist, had developed a somewhat unusual but benign cardiac arrhythmia. His heart skipped beats, some times more frequently than at other times, but every day and often throughout the day. Although he knew his condition was not dangerous-at least so he had been told by two cardiologists-he remained very worried. He took his pulse dozens of times each day even though the amount of medication prescribed for him was no different whether he had a lot of missed beats or only a few. In other words, counting his heart beats provided no information useful for managing his condition. And he knew this too. When I asked him to stop taking his pulse, he replied, "I'll try."

Such a response implies a complicated point of view: first of all, taken literally, it means he did not feel certain that he could stop! Secondly, he was obviously not entirely convinced that stopping would really help him, or he would have determined to do so no matter how difficult it seemed. His subsequent course was typical. In fits and starts he did cut down on the frequency of taking his pulse. He did not stop entirely until his cardiologist agreed that it was a good idea. A few weeks later, he reported himself as "markedly improved."

Stop checking for only a few weeks, and you will see for yourself that your mind will wander away from thoughts of illness, real or imaginary, and back to work and family and having fun, and all the other mundane matters that ordinarily occupy our lives.

2. Do not ask for reassurance.

I start with the assumption that we live our lives most effectively and happily when we know what is real. The more we know about the real dangers of the world, the better able we are to cope with them and the less we are likely to be afraid unnecessarily. As far as I can remember, most of the worries I have had, usually concerns about my health or the health of members of my family, have been unjustified. Most of the terrible things I have been able to imagine have never come to pass. What we should be seeking, health worriers in particular, is to learn the truth about ourselves and our circumstances. Most of the time, the truth is reassuring. Even when the news is seemingly bad, there is often some saving grace discernible- some sort of cure, for instance. When we are, in fact, sick, we want to know about it in order to take measures to heal ourselves. When we are not truly sick - even though we may have physical symptoms - we want to know that too so we can put thoughts of these symptoms to one side and go on with our lives.

Health worriers would not quarrel with this point of view. Some, of course, are afraid of doctors and stay away from them even when they are ill; but they know they are not being sensible at those times. They understand that postponing these visits is endangering their health. The majority, however, go to doctors at the first sign of being sick, or before; and then, usually unsatisfied, they go from one doctor to another. If asked, they would say that they are looking for answers.

They want to know if they are seriously sick, or not. They want to know if any remedial measures need to be taken. They want to know if they are safe. Listening to their questions, though, a doctor may well conclude that they are unwilling to take "yes" for an answer.

"This pain starts in the back and goes into the groin. Do you think it could be the sciatic nerve?

"No, it's just a muscle spasm."

"Well, it starts right here on the side."

"Don't worry, it's just a muscle spasm."

"Well, isn't it true that you can get pain shooting down right here sometimes from sciatica?"

"Yes. Sometimes. But then you have signs of pain when you stretch the nerve. And it's not quite in that location anyway."

"So, it <u>could</u> be sciatica?"

Although such a patient may think she is looking for the truth and is certainly, she would say, looking for reassurance, she seems to be unwilling to settle for either. She starts with the conviction that she has a particular illness, which she is especially afraid of, and then distorts whatever the doctor says until it conforms with that prejudice. Yet she does not <u>want</u> to think she really has that condition. Not consciously or unconsciously. She simply hears what she expects to hear. What she <u>wants</u> to hear is something that will unequivocally expunge any doubts she may have; and no such explanation, however unambiguous, is possible.

Another patient:

"I feel worse. I can't sleep or eat anything. This medicine is making me feel worse."

"It's not the medicine. It's the depression. You remember, you felt the same way before taking the medicine. Every day you said you felt worse."

"Can I stop the medicine?"

"No. You will feel better in three to four weeks. Otherwise you'll feel the same way you felt these last six months."

The next day.

"I feel worse. I can't eat or sleep. And I have headaches. I think it's the medicine."

"Keep taking the medicine. You're going to feel bad for another three weeks. Then you'll feel much better."

"I didn't feel this bad before I started the medicine."

"Yes, you did. You said you did."

"Can't the medicine cause headaches and nausea?"

"Just keep taking the medicine for another three weeks. Then you'll feel better."

"I looked it up; the medicine can cause these symptoms."

"Please keep taking it. No kidding, you'll feel better in about three weeks.

The next day:

"I think this medicine is making me feel sick. I feel weird walking down the street."

"You'll be fine. Just like the last couple of times you got depressed."

"How long is it going to take?"

"About three weeks."

This telephone conversation was repeated 15 times over the next three weeks and a couple of times again in the following week since the anti-depressants took, on this occasion, a full month to work.

Why did this woman call again and again? Surely not to elicit more information, for the conversation took on a stereotyped, scripted form in which each person said only what he or she had said during each previous conversation. She was looking for "reassurance," she would have said. Her family called her "clinging" or "needy."

I think it was the telephone call itself that mattered to her. She too had a preconceived idea about what was making her ill-in this case the medicine itself; but the reason she called had little to do with sorting out her treatment and more to do with her emotional state. It was her feeling of being misunderstood, unattended to, and alone that made her call.

In the case of someone who is acutely depressed, the ritual of calling is justified; and a caring physician will listen patiently. It is for a circumscribed period only and is not likely to worsen the patient's dependence or aggravate her health anxiety. But, in general, responding with the same answers to the same question accomplishes nothing and tends to center the patient's attention more fixedly on her, or his, symptoms.

Imagine a scene in a doctor's office where a patient has just been examined for a complaint that does not seem significant in the doctor's eye. The illness, which is real enough, does not match up with the finite number of medical diseases listed in a medical textbook. Perhaps the patient has a nondescript pain, or a minor gastrointestinal complaint, or sees lights when he looks off to one side. The doctor tells the patient that there is nothing seriously the matter with him; but the patient persists - as in the examples above - to ask further questions, especially "Why?" "Why do I have this nondescript pain?"

The doctor does not really know why. This particular nondescript pain is not <u>important</u> enough to have made it into the medical textbook. In other words, it is not of a sort that is likely to worsen in severity or spread to other parts of the body, or linger, for then it would have appeared in the medical textbook. The doctor, therefore, can answer in one of 2 ways:

1. (Honestly) "I don't know why you're having this pain; but I expect it to go away."

Such an answer is not likely to satisfy the health worrier. (See above.)

2. (Making up an answer.) "You may have sprained something."

These answers are likely to be taken more seriously than they deserve. The health worrier is likely to worry about spraining himself further. And, of course, whatever the doctor says, the health worrier considers more serious possibilities.

"Are you sure?" the patient asks.

This question is one of a number to which people cannot respond intelligently or convincingly. "Do you love me?" is another.

The doctor can reply in one of three ways:

1. (Honestly) "No, I'm not sure, because medicine is not an exact science, and it is not possible ever to be sure."

This is surely not the reassurance the health worrier was looking for.

2. (Blurring the truth) "Yes, I'm sure. Go home and stop worrying."

This response is not reassuring because the patient knows full well that medicine is not an exact science, and it is not possible ever to be sure.

3. (Changing the subject) "Try to relax a little."

This response is foolish and embarrasses both the patient and the doctor.

Some rules for patients:

1. If you want to, make a list of questions ahead of time to ask the doctor. This annoys some doctors but makes sense to me. If you are very anxious during the visit, you will forget to ask about something that worries you and, then, later on, will agonize about whether or not you should risk bothering the doctor by calling him or her on the telephone.

2. Ask the right questions. Do not ask whether cancer can cause your nondescript pain because the answer is "yes." Ask whether the nondescript pain you have is likely to be caused by cancer. That is what you really want to know. Cancer can sometimes cause:

> Headache.
> Runny nose.
> Swollen glands.
> Constipation.
> Skin rashes and probably every other
> physical symptom.

This does not mean you should worry about cancer every time you get a headache or a runny nose. If you are worried, reasonably or not, about a particular serious disease, ask the doctor if there is a likelihood that you have that disease. Do not ask theoretical questions about the disease itself Do not ask questions such as "What makes you think so?" which lead to complicated medical textbook-type explanations and which are not likely to be understandable or convincing.

3. Do not ask repetitive questions or rhetorical questions.

Repeated a number of times in the space of five minutes:

"So you don't think it's anything serious?"

"So you think I'll be okay?"

"And the pain itself, that doesn't mean anything, is that what you said? So, I'll be all right in a couple of weeks, you said?"

The replies to these questions do not vary from one minute to the next and, most likely not from one day to the next. Prodding the doctor repeatedly in this way is no different than checking one's pulse over and over again and has the same disadvantages. It is compulsive in character. It elicits no new information. Also, in its own small way, it is annoying and interferes with the doctor-patient relationship.

"Are you sure?"

"Is that what you really think?"

These are rhetorical questions only and do not advance your understanding of your medical problems.

Do not ask your family their opinion of your medical problem. They do not know any more about it than you do. Do not ask them if you feel feverish to their touch, if your eyes are bloodshot, if you look pale, or if you seem to them to be getting better or worse. They are likely to say something encouraging which you will not believe because you know they care about you and are likely to say something encouraging when they do not really mean it. Then you will be reduced to asking them if they really mean it, and they will say they really mean it whether or not they really mean it.

If a medical consultation is likely to be emotionally charged, bring along a family member. When patients are frightened, they cannot hear accurately what their doctors are telling them. Naturally. Sometimes it is necessary to schedule a second appointment simply to go over the same issues again when the patient is calmer. Health worriers, of course, tend to be more frightened than ordinary patients. When they mis-hear, it is usually in a particular direction: things sound worse than they really are. Often patients return to their doctors' offices asking them to elaborate on a diagnosis the doctors never made. Worse, sometimes health worriers are afraid to return to their doctors' offices and so remain convinced that the doctors have given them bad news when no such thing has happened.

One way of avoiding these misunderstanding is to bring along someone else who can listen to the doctor more dispassionately. Such a person, usually a family member, can correct the sometimes striking distortions that characterize the patient's impression of what was said. If the patient begins to wander off into irrelevance, the family member can sometimes help to focus the consultation.

What the patient needs to know is what is the matter with him or her medically (insofar as it is possible to say at that time,) what needs to be done to investigate the condition further, what treatment should be instituted, and what complication of that treatment should be anticipated, and, finally, what is the likely outcome.

4. Do not encourage the doctor to perform laboratory tests or other investigative procedures that he does not suggest on his own initiative. Do not encourage the doctor to prescribe specific treatments that he has not thought to recommend.

Certain tests, like the M.R.I. (magnetic resonance imaging) have captured the imagination of the public. Painless and harmless, these tests allow a physician to peer inside any part of the body and visualize soft tissues in addition to the bony structures apparent to x-rays. Other tests, such as biopsies, have the reputation of revealing definitely whether a particular illness is present or not. This promise is not always fulfilled. Because health worriers often want to know definitely whether they are truly sick or not, what exactly is making them sick, and just exactly how sick they may be, they encourage their physicians to use these magical tests, and others, to get an answer once and for all. But unequivocal answers are not within reach for reasons mentioned previously. For one thing, many tests become positive only at critical times. For example, certain tests for pregnancy are not positive at the beginning of pregnancy, become positive later on and then become negative again still later on! Most doctors are not inclined to pursue an illusory and unnecessary certainty. They may not want to put the patient through tests which are, even in the case of an M.R.I, uncomfortable at best and anxiety-provoking. And expensive. But most doctors are responsive ultimately to their patients demands. Doctors have referred patients to me complaining that in the course of their treatment they had undergone medical workups costing hundreds of thousands of dollars "for no reason at all," as if they, the doctors themselves, bore no responsibility for ordering the tests. The doctor is a trained expert, and the patient is not; but very often it is the patient who decides in the end what tests will be performed. What follows inevitably are more tests that deepen the patient's anxieties without ever giving definitive answers.

Similarly, prescribing drugs appropriately requires a sophisticated judgment about many relevant factors. A partial list:

1. The nature of the illness for which the drug is being prescribed. Is it a serious condition, possibly life-threatening? Are the symptoms it causes very severe? Untreated, is it likely to be disabling? Is it likely to remit without drugs? Depression, for example, usually goes away even untreated somewhere between six months and a year and a half after it begins.

2. The presence of other illnesses which might complicate treatment. A drug which improves one condition may aggravate another.

3. The effect that a particular treatment may have on subsequent diagnostic tests. For example, antibiotics prescribed prematurely for a sore throat will invalidate the results of a subsequent throat culture.
4. The effectiveness of one drug, more or less, compared to another.
5. The need for certain drugs to be monitored closely with blood tests. There are many such drugs.
6. The potential of a drug for abuse. Does it cause a high? Is it habit-forming?
7. The means by which the body eliminates the drug. Is the drug detoxified and excreted through the lungs, the liver or the kidney, any one of which can be diseased? Is the drug excreted through the skin, causing body odor?
8. The route of administration of the drug. Must it be given by injection or can it be taken orally, or rectally? Does it have to be given in multiple doses, leaving more room for error?
9. Effects on a pregnancy. Does the drug cause fetal malformations when given to pregnant women? Is it passed along to an infant through breast-feeding?
10. The toxicity of the drug. Does it cause many side-effects? How troublesome are they likely to be? Are there likely to be long-range side-effects not yet known? Because of this possibility, drugs that have been prescribed to many people over a period of many years may be safer than newer drugs.
11. The half-life of the drug. Is the drug likely to accumulate in the body? The therapeutic index, that is the margin between the therapeutic dose and a toxic dose, is also important.
12. The reliability of the patient. Is the patient in such a state of mind that he or she is likely to take too much or too little medicine, accidentally or on purpose?
13. The age, weight and sex of the patient, all of which may affect dose.

And so on.

Given all these consideration, is it reasonable for a patient to have an opinion as to which drug would be best to treat his or her medical condition?

I was drafted into the army many years ago and was stationed in a hospital in Nuremberg, Germany. I served as a psychiatrist, but like all the other doctors, I took night call to see medical emergencies. One evening a colonel brought in his 7 year old son to be examined. The boy had a cold and was coughing a little. I told the officer that his son was going to be fine and did not require any medication.

"I brought him here to get some cough medicine," he replied.

"He doesn't need any cough medicine. Besides, it's not really a good idea since he once had an attack of asthma, or something like asthma."

"I want him to have cough medicine. He's coughing; and I always give him cough medicine."

"Look, I'm not going to give him any cough medicine because I think it's a bad idea. If you want to check with the pediatrician tomorrow, that's fine."

"You know, if I don't get it from you, I'm going right out to the nearest German drug store and get it there."

"Great. You do whatever you want to do. But I'm the doctor, and I'm supposed to use my best medical judgment; and my best medical judgment is that your son is better off without cough medicine. And I'm not going to give it to him!"

Exit the colonel in a huff, pulling his son along by the arm.

Now, suppose I had been a civilian pediatrician trying to maintain a private practice. Would I have prescribed the cough medicine? Sure, I would have. And the parent would not have had to ask me three times. The livelihood of a doctor depends on his ability to satisfy his customers. I would not have prescribed poison to the kid, just to please his father; but probably the cough medicine would not

176

have been harmful. Very likely, judging from my experience of other doctors, I would have convinced myself that this particular cough medicine might conceivably help, given these particular circumstances, parental attitudes, etc. Doctors, like everybody else, are subject to this sort of pressure. For one thing, like everyone else, they like to please.

Patients often want to come away from a doctor's office with something in hand to make them better, or feel better, at least. Good medical advice is not enough. As a result, whole classes of drugs are prescribed when they ought not to be. These include cough medicines, sleeping pills, laxatives, tranquilizers, pain relievers, antibiotics and others. Most of the time patients are no worse off as a result; but sometimes they definitely are. Pseudomembranous colitis is a very serious bacterial infection of the intestines caused by the prolonged use of antibiotics. It is relatively uncommon. As a psychiatrist, I have only come across three cases, all of which required multiple prolonged hospitalizations. In each case, the antibiotic causing the condition had been prescribed unnecessarily!

As a patient, you have a right, even an obligation, to be involved in decisions concerning your medical care. Often a physician will present you with alternatives from which you can reasonably choose one or another. I, myself, after presenting the respective pros and cons, offer depressed patients the choice between two different classes of anti-depressants. One anti-depressant tends to make the patient gain weight, the other tends to interfere with sex. About 90% of patients, women mostly, choose to put their sex life at risk rather than risk getting fat. But you should not recommend drugs for your physician to prescribe to you because you read about it in a magazine. For similar reasons, you should not on your own initiative take medicines that have been prescribed for your spouse. These drugs are likely to be out of date and, consequently, potentially harmful. They may be harmful for other reasons.

Chapter Nine: The Nightmare Fantasy

Health anxiety is by definition an irrational fear, that is, an exaggerated and unrealistic fear. The way to overcome any such fear is by confronting it. If the danger is seen to be unreal, the fear of it will disappear. Psychotherapists are always trying to get their patients to confront the various irrational fears that constrain their lives, whether they are something specific such as the fear of snakes or more general like the fear of success. Certain fears turn out to be realistic, in which case measures can be taken to lessen the risk. More commonly, the fears are based upon misconceptions of one sort or another; and these will be dispelled with repeated exposure to the feared situation. So much is easier said than done, however.

There are two problems. The most obvious is the patients' unwillingness or, perhaps, inability to do scary things. A person afraid of bridges will surely get over the fear if he or she spends enough time on bridges. However, the brief time spent crossing a particular bridge every once in a while is not enough because the ride is unpleasant from beginning to end. There is not time enough to calm down. On the other hand, someone afraid of the water, but willing to slosh around in a pool all afternoon every afternoon for a summer, will inevitably learn to feel comfortable and will probably learn to swim in the bargain, even without instruction. There are some people so afraid of snakes that they are afraid of leaving their apartment buildings. If they were willing to spend a couple of days in a room with snakes slithering all over the floor, they would without question get over their fear of snakes. But how does a therapist get someone terrified of snakes into a room full of snakes? It is impossible.

Successful treatment has to go a little bit at a time. This process is not only inherently unpleasant, but also it is time-con-suming. The patient reads about snakes, then looks at pictures of snakes, then carries around a toy snake, then looks at snakes in a glass cage. Looking at a snake in a cage is really boring. Usually it takes a while to figure out if the snake is dead or alive. The next step involves getting closer and closer to the snake, then watching someone else hold a real snake and then, finally, ending up actually handling the snake. This kind of treatment is called desensitization. It always works if someone can be motivated to spend the time to do it. It does not matter whether or not the patient undertakes this process hopefully or resentfully. Most patients respond to a sympathetic and reasoned approach by a therapist. Some other patients may only be motivated by the threat of their condition getting worse otherwise. The only thing that matters is the patient's willingness to confront his or her irrational fear systematically and over a long enough period of time to allow that fear to dissipate.

So much is straightforward in principle, however difficult it may be to implement in practice. The fear of snakes is overcome by confronting snakes; and when treatment is successful the fear of snakes is gone. But there are other irrational fears that are not so concrete and specific as the fear of snakes. And, out of this circumstance, comes the second problem in treatment. <u>Desensitization only works when it is clear exactly what the patient is afraid of.</u>

Consider two different women who are obsessed with the possibility of developing breast cancer. Very likely they have many overlapping fears, but it may turn out, usually after considerable probing, that one is primarily afraid of mutilating surgery and the other is afraid of the pain of cancer. Talking to the first woman endlessly about the details of dying from cancer will not help her overcome her fear, and talking to the second woman at whatever length about the details of a mastectomy will not help her overcome her fear. <u>It is not usually clear just what the health worrier is afraid of when he or she reports a fear of cancer, or a heart attack, or even, simply a fear of dying.</u> Some people, for instance, are afraid of dying, but not of being dead; others are afraid of death but not of dying.

A woman who was afraid of flying said she had no fear of death itself but was afraid of those agonizing moments after the wing of the airplane cracks and falls off, and the plane plummets out of the sky. She was also afraid of cancer, but not of dying. She was afraid of the awful chore of saying good-bye to her children after her doctor tells her she has only three months to live.

Another woman was not afraid of the process of dying, which she imagined to be like falling asleep, but of what she imagined death to be like. She pictured herself buried underground in a coffin on a cold, deserted hillside. Another such woman was afraid of spending an eternity in hell because of sexual indiscretions she had committed 40 years before. I told her there was a 10 year statute of limitations on such crimes, and if she had not died during that time she could not be held accountable; but she was in no mood to be jollied up.

The particular individual concerns of the health worrier must be addressed if there is any hope of the condition going away. These are not usually one or two but rather an overlapping hierarchy of fears. They have to be taken up in the order in which they present themselves to the patient. Contrary to what he or she may say, initial worries usually have nothing to do either with death or dying.

For example, a patient may be preoccupied, first of all, with her panic attacks. She asks: "What if my heart goes so fast I have a heart attack; and I'm miles away from the nearest hospital?" She pictures to herself a scene in which she lies helpless on the ground, alone, or surrounded by uncaring strangers. That is the fantasy that comes to her mind. If pressed about what would happen next, she might very well say that she could die, but that is not usually what she thinks about. She thinks only of the "what if...", not of the "well, then..." that comes after. Coming to terms with death in the abstract would not help her. She has to learn that a panic attack cannot cause a heart attack, and that most heart attacks do not leave a person writhing helplessly on the ground. She needs to understand that most strangers would come to her aid if she did indeed have a heart attack. She needs to confront her particular fears. If over the course of treatment she loses her fear of panic, she may still retain her fear of a heart attack. She may be preoccupied then with a different fantasy. Lying in bed she feels her heart skip a beat or suddenly beat very quickly; and she thinks "what if my heart stops altogether?" To overcome this somewhat related fear, she needs to know that the premature auricular or ventricular contractions she notices when she is resting quietly in bed are normal and, like the tachycardia she always feels when she gets frightened, do not lead to heart attacks even over a period of many years. If this particular fear dissipates, as it often does, she may find herself haunted by still another thought. "Suppose that mole I've been looking at on my back has gotten a little bigger…" She may not be thinking just about the implications of developing a malignant melanoma, but also about the sick, terrified feeling she will have running her fingers back and forth across the mole, and the worried look on her husband's face as he examines the mole. She may be imagining her anxiety growing minute by minute until she sees her doctor – and that the doctor may not be available. Her fear is not just a single thought but a complex scenario that is played out over and over again in her mind. She may have other lurking fears that are always in the background: "What if I turn on the television and there is a program on about leukemia?" "What if my sister gets bad news from her doctor?" "What if I read about someone my age getting ovarian cancer and I start worrying all the time about that?"

Probably the nightmare fantasy that bothers most patients when they start treatment for health anxiety is a scene they imagine taking place in their doctor's office.

Doctor: Sit down, please. There's something I want to talk to you about. I don't want you to worry. (A signal to start worrying.) But I noticed a small lump I'm a little concerned about. It's probably nothing, but I want to order a few tests.

Patient: Well. . . .could it be cancer?

Doctor: Let's just wait. There's no point in worrying about things that could be or might be.

It is the fear of just such an encounter that keeps some health worriers from ever visiting a doctor. If the patient can be desensitized to this sort of encounter, additional fears become apparent: the imagined scene where the patient is wheeled away from his family into an operating room; the scene where the doctor says "we think we got it all," but probably did not; all the occasions later on when the patient has to go for further tests to see if the cancer has spread; the chemotherapy and the resultant vomiting and loss of hair; the time still later on when the patient has wasted away and become ugly.

A common fear is of hospitalization. One patient may imagine tubes being passed into every orifice. Another imagines the end of visiting hours when a spouse leaves the hospital to go shopping, and the patient is left alone. Another may be terrified by the pain she imagines is an inevitable consequence of terminal cancer. Almost everyone, I think, imagines unsympathetic doctors who determine treatment arbitrarily without regard to the patient's wishes and who cannot be reached at night. No one expects nurses to respond when called. When all these fears are surmounted, there may remain the fear of dying. Some people see themselves as helpless, unable to talk. Others see themselves as alone, perhaps in the middle of the night. <u>In no sense is the fear of dying more fundamental than these other fears</u>. It is not that fear that underlies all the other fears. In fact, there are other fears that are more fundamental and that do in some real sense underlie the fear of dying.

A young woman who had just completed her medical training had worked her way through a number of fears similar to those described above. Finally, towards the end of treatment she began contemplating her own death. She saw herself having failed all medical treatment, dead, lying in a coffin surrounded by her family. When this scene presented itself in her mind's eye, she began crying. In her fantasizing she realizes she will never live to practice her profession or to have children. She will never see again all those family gathered around her. What, then, was she afraid of? Not just the fear of dying, although that too. She was afraid that all the things that she had always wanted and worked for would be lost forever. And she was afraid of being alone. Forever. These are fears that grow out of life's experiences. Not everyone shares these fears; and something can be done about them.

For most people the fear of death is a metaphor, a symbolic representation of two other primitive fears:

1. The fear of being alone, and
2. The fear of being helpless.

Often, patients imagine themselves continuing on somehow even after they are dead! They picture themselves buried underground in the cold and dark, unable to see anything, unable to move, and horribly alone, forever. These fears may have roots going back to childhood. They may reflect times when as children they were ignored or made to feel useless. But now that they are grown, if they live in a way that is valuable in the eyes of others, if they share their life with friends and family, and especially with children, those fears will diminish. And, along the way, the fear of dying too.

The range of specific fears that can become part of a health anxiety is large. Here are some of them:

1. The fear in the event of death of leaving one's children behind helpless or feeling abandoned.
2. The fear of having a child kidnapped if one were to have a sudden heart attack in a public place.
3. The fear of being immobilized suddenly by a stroke and unable to get to a telephone to call for help.
4. The fear of chemotherapy, or medication in general, or surgery, or simply of being examined medically.
5. The fear of being ignored by friends or family who are too upset to spend any time visiting.

6. The fear of being forgotten in the event of death.
7. The fear that a fatal illness may already be present, but lurking undiagnosed.
8. The fear that fear itself may be causing irrevocable long-term bodily damage such as heart disease.
9. The superstitious fear that worrying about a particular disease (or after a while not worrying about that disease) will cause that disease.
10. The fear of degenerating into some ugly and repellent state.
11. The fear of a doctor taking away a favorite medication.
12. The fear of catching somebody else's illness or even someone else's fear of a particular illness.
13. The fear of finding a new spot or lump, or finding it to be bigger.
14. The fear of germs or contamination.
15. The fear of prolonged illness or catastrophic illnesses, such as becoming a quadriplegic.
16. The fear of particular disabilities, such as going blind.
17. The fear of having life support removed by well-meaning or not so well-meaning relatives.
18. The fear of being buried alive.
19. The fear of hearing upsetting medical news.
20. The fear of being too far away from a hospital to receive emergency medical care.
21. The fear of one's children developing a painful or fatal condition.
22. The fear of being pitied by everyone.

And, or course, the fear of many particular diseases: brain tumors, leukemia, aneurysms, AIDS, ovarian and pancreatic cancer, malignant melanoma, heart attacks, multiple sclerosis and so on. These conditions have some elements in common:

1. They may lurk in the body without giving signs of their presence.

2. They tend to appear suddenly and sometimes with devastating effect.
3. They are largely incurable, and often fatal.

Some of these fears, such as the fear of hospitals or needles, are concrete and can be confronted directly. But some, like the fear of becoming helpless or useless, are a kind of vague, formless dread. How does one practice coping with them? How does someone confront an existential fear?

There is always a bridge nearby to practice on for someone afraid of bridges. The local pet store has snakes for snake phobias. But how does someone confront an abstraction like the fear of dying? We cannot give someone cancer just for a little while so that person can get used to it. We are not prepared to operate on someone in order to help them get over their fear of anesthesia.

Many years ago, when less was understood about phobias, treatment involved patients confronting mental images of the phobic situation or object they were avoiding, while they were at the same time attempting to relax. Instead of confronting snakes or their equivalent, the patients were told to <u>imagine</u> snakes. When those images became less threatening after awhile, they were told to imagine the snake coming closer. And still try to relax. It turned out that desensitization did not require being in a relaxed state. It also turns out, as one might expect, that confronting real snakes works better as a treatment than picturing an imaginary snake. But, even so, just thinking of snakes did indeed considerably lessen the fear of snakes in many people, especially if they were in general sensitive and imaginative. Health worriers are precisely that kind of person. Hearing about someone else's heart attack, they can experience chest pain directly over their own heart, although true cardiac pain is experienced midline in the chest and not over the left side. They can see a rash which is invisible to a dermatologist. Women often find breast lumps that were not present the day before. And they can vividly imagine dying without actually dying and without any realistic threat of dying. Instead of thinking suddenly and briefly these terrifying thoughts, health worriers need to dwell on them purposely, if they can be persuaded to do so, long enough for the panicky feeling to wear off.

It is not very hard for someone afraid of bridges to believe that if he or she spends enough time on bridges the fear will go away. But very few people who are afraid of dying can accept readily the idea that that fear will go away if they spend enough time mulling it over. In fact, they would say that they spend too much time already obsessed by these thoughts. Actually, what they do is, suddenly, without particular provocation, think these thoughts repeatedly, all day long, but never for any length of time and never thinking them though. Every time the thought comes to them unbidden they have a sinking, sick feeling which they turn away from as soon as they can only to have it return forcibly a little while later. The job of the therapist is to marshal his or her influence and authority and whatever trust has been built up in the therapeutic relationship to encourage the patient to try this difficult and somewhat counterintuitive treatment long enough to see if it works. For surely it does work.

Dispelling the Nightmare Fantasy

First, it must be determined just which particular health worry is haunting the patient currently. It is more likely to be an encounter in the doctor's office than the thought of dying. That scene should be expanded and embellished with as much realistic detail as possible. It should be as real as a scene in the theater. A therapist playing the part of the doctor can act out this role so that the patient becomes distinctly uncomfortable. Ultimately, as with the treatment of any phobia, the patient must decide how much exposure is tolerable and how much is so uncomfortable it cannot be managed initially. But the therapist must make the scene so vivid the patient understands what is required. The patient is <u>supposed</u> to feel uncomfortable. If someone afraid of bridges walks immediately onto a bridge <u>comfortably</u>, then the fear that the person expressed is not really a fear of bridges. If the nightmare fantasy the patient conjures up does not produce any distress, then some critical element of the fantasy is missing. Once an appropriate version of the nightmare fantasy is fixed upon, the patient is asked to visualize himself or herself in that situation - for an entire hour at a time. More specifically, the patient is encouraged to put off worrying if possible until that particular hour of the day. During that hour the patient should try as much as possible to imagine that fantasy becoming real. <u>At the same time, at intervals the patient should remind himself or herself just how unlikely is the event being considered.</u> Also, the patient is invited to consider the "well, then... which should follow the "what if..."

"Well, if the lump is bad enough to biopsy, still the doctor says it is unlikely to be cancer."

"Well, if the lump turns out to be cancer, the doctor says that we got it early enough to cure."

"Well, if the lump is too big to remove completely, this kind of cancer doesn't metastasize. So, even if it comes back, it won't kill me."

And so on. These somewhat comforting thoughts should be based on the truth, of course. They are a legitimate aspect of the otherwise dreadful situation the patient fears.

If the patient can be persuaded to undertake this seemingly perverse mental exercise for an entire hour for even only a few days in a row, the sick, frightened and awful feeling begins noticeably to disappear. The unthinkable becomes thinkable. Very quickly a thought that was terrifying becomes boring, and the exercise of confronting the nightmare fantasy becomes simply another routine chore. The patient's attention begins to wander and can be kept focused sometimes only by writing out in narrative form the exact details of fantasy: the concerned look on the physician's face, the telephone call that interrupts his or her comments, the complicated plan about what to do next, even the details of how the office looks and sounds. The more real the better. And then, when this particular scene becomes drab and uninteresting, it must be changed to something more upsetting! Perhaps the next nightmare to get used to is waiting for the laboratory report - or the scene in the doctor's office when the doctor announces reluctantly that the biopsy has come back positive. Or a scene in the hospital. Or a scene with family gathered tearfully about a hospital sickbed.

It is important to start with the nightmare fantasy foremost in the patient's mind and then proceed to other fears that may not be immediately apparent. Sometimes the person who seems primarily to be afraid of a heart attack is really afraid that her children will wander away if she falls insensible to the ground in the middle of a department store. Someone else may be afraid of going crazy only because he is afraid of screaming and making a fool of himself. Often these fears, once they are articulated, can be addressed directly. Those afraid of their orphaned children becoming impoverished after they die can make financial arrangements that will guarantee that not happening. Those afraid of being helpless in the face of a doctor's whims can develop a relationship with a sympathetic doctor to whom they can explain their concerns.

It is not uncommon for people to say that what they are "really" afraid of is the uncontrollable pain of terminal cancer. Certainly, pain is a common feature of terminal illness, and too many patients do suffer severe pain; but there is no good reason for this to happen. There are very effective medicines available now for managing even very severe pain. Such a person can usually be reassured with a proper, sufficiently detailed, explanation. Many times the specific nightmare fantasy a patient has is completely unrealistic - a unicorn. The patient may be afraid of becoming totally paralyzed from a minor, inconsequential disease, and here too, a simple explanation that no one has taken the time previously to offer may calm the health worrier.

Sometimes, the nightmare fantasy has to do with an uncertain family relationship. One man imagined himself dying in a hospital with neither his children nor his wife willing to visit him. Such an idea may need to be treated in a family context. Many such fears are essentially a variant on the thought of abandonment. They stem from early experiences and need to be understood in those terms. Sometimes the fear of abandonment extends past the point of death to an imaginary time and place where the person is buried under an unattended patch of grass, unvisited and forgotten.

It should be noted again that patients who have been treated for cancer or for some other potentially fatal disease are not usually troubled by nightmare fantasies, at least of that particular illness. Every day represents 24 hours of practicing confronting that illness, and it loses its sting quickly. Only when they go for a further check up or when there is laboratory evidence that their disease is worsening do they get upset.

Some people are so anxious about so many different things that they are said to be suffering from a generalized anxiety disorder: the "anxiety disease." It is easy to rationalize, therefore, taking anti-anxiety agents. They are among the most commonly prescribed drugs in the world. I think it is often more to the point, however, to deal with these various fears one after the other. Many of them, such as the nightmare fantasies, are irrational. And many of them overlap. Health worriers usually have particular fears of drugs, doctors, medical tests, diseases and even sometimes a fear of looking at or touching their own bodies. It often seems that as one fear disappears another rises to take its place. But still, with proper treatment, many of these fears disappear one after the other forever. And some others return only in a milder form when something happens in the real world to trigger them once again. At such a time learning as much as possible about the medical danger, if it is real, will allow that person to take measures to minimize the risk to health. If the fear is irrational, it will disappear. Immersing oneself in the details of a nightmare fantasy is one way of learning the truth, in this case learning about the truth of one's own feelings. People will become accustomed to any unchanging condition. The feeling of dread in particular cannot last in any familiar situation unless something truly dangerous happens. People calm down eventually, even those who seem to worry incessantly and perpetually.

Chapter Ten: Insomnia and Fear of Drugs

Among the Bad Ideas mentioned previously, two are worth special note. First, the concern health worriers are likely to have about ordinary bodily functions, such as eating and sleeping, is important because it can lead to a disruption of those functions. Second, misplaced concerns they have about taking medication – almost any kind of medication – makes it difficult for them to deal properly with illness when they do, in fact, get sick.

Bad Ideas about eating, sleeping and elimination

These sum to the idea that any deviation from the usual is a deviation from normal.

First of all, health worriers worry typically that they may not be eating an optimum diet. It is not unusual-in fact, it is appropriate - to recognize a connection between nutrition and health; but while ordinary people manage effortlessly to eat well enough, health worriers can become preoccupied by their diet. It is one example among many of health worriers focusing on a legitimate concern and taking it to an unreasonable extreme. They worry about getting sick if they fast. They may drink 8 or 9 glasses of water a day, even when they are not thirsty, in order to eliminate "toxins" from their bodies that are eliminated just as well by eating and drinking normally. Of course, they find support for these ideas by reading uncritically published articles of one sort or another. A few misguided individuals drink to such great excess that they wash too much sodium out of their system. As a result, every few years I admit someone to the hospital with an organic psychosis due simply to a low blood sodium. Certain other extreme diets recommended for health reasons are so dangerous that they threaten life in addition to health. Commonly, health worriers think their children do not eat enough. Pressure to get the children to eat more and to eat properly can make mealtimes miserable. If eating "good" foods is required, these foods will seem less desirable. Adult eating disorders are in part a product of these experiences.

The fact is: like most animals, human beings naturally eat a more or less reasonable diet. A caveat: It is true that for various reasons too many people have become fat. Being thin is healthier. But it is not important to eat properly today, or tomorrow, or even all this week. Over the course of a lifetime diet makes a real difference, but it should not be a matter of desperate concern every day. As indicated in various places in this book, taking extra vitamins may be advisable. There is no advantage in eating "organic" foods. The amounts of carcinogens, and anti-carcinogens, present in all foods dwarfs the amounts added by using chemical fertilizers or insecticides. Except when employed in a grossly inappropriate manner, they do not represent a health hazard. Of course, a whole industry has grown up to capitalize on this misconception; and adherents hold to it with a religious fervor.

The process of elimination is not worthy of a great deal of attention. There is no medical information that can be obtained from viewing urine in a toilet bowl. Urine that is concentrated and very yellow is just as good as pale. Health worriers, and others too, worry too much about their stool. Too cylindrical, one patient told me. Constipation may be unpleasant, but it is not a cause of ill health. Severe constipation may require medical, or even surgical, management, but occasional constipation is likely to be a function of changing diet or stress and requires no treatment. The most common cause of recurrent constipation is excessive reliance on laxatives. In just such a way an exaggerated concern about a symptom can make that symptom worse. Another symptom that comes frequently solely from worrying about it too much is insomnia.

Insomnia

The most common cause for insomnia is pain, usually from disorders that affect older people. The medical management of insomnia in these cases is the management of the underlying disease. Another under-appreciated cause of insomnia is depression, which is treated successfully by anti-depressant drugs. In these cases sleeping medicines have only limited effectiveness. In fact, patients use sleeping medicines as a rule for periods much longer than is usually recommended by their manufacturers. Just as the use of laxatives leads to chronic constipation, the continual use of hypnotics-sleep-inducing drugs - worsens insomnia. After only a few weeks of use, dependency appears. Stopping the drug then leads to delayed onset of sleep and interrupted sleep - and sometimes nightmares. The nightmares can be so troubling that some people stay on these drugs indefinitely, just to avoid them.

A principle cause of insomnia, however, is the Bad Idea many health worriers hold, to wit: that a good night's sleep, every night, is critically important to health and to their day-to-day functioning.

"Unless I get a good night's sleep, I'm no good the next day."

Or "I get more panic attacks after a sleepless night."

Or "If I don't sleep one night, I get sick with something."

Somebody who goes to bed with the desperate thought that he, or she, must sleep in order to perform well - let's say give a good business presentation the next day - is not likely to fall asleep readily. If sleep is delayed for a half-hour, that person may become too upset to sleep at all. Similarly, if someone wakes up anxiously at 2:10, 2:20 and 2:30 A.M. and then again at 4: 10, 4:20 and 4:30 A.M., that person is likely to think he, or she, has not slept at all. Getting worried in the middle of the night is not conducive to falling back to sleep.

The fact is: that the only consequence likely to result from missing a night's sleep is being sleepy the next day. As medical interns demonstrate all the time, important intellectual tasks are not compromised by going without sleep. The ability to perform rote tasks, such as bookkeeping, is affected adversely by prolonged sleeplessness; but someone engaged in an important task, such as giving a business presentation, will do fine. Panic attacks do not come from sleeplessness; but they do stem, in part, from the expectation of getting panicky. So, people who on the basis of their past experiences expect to get panicky after a poor night's sleep may very well get panicky in that setting, just as others habitually get panicky after having a sugary meal or at dusk. It is very difficult to convince such a person that sleep has no intrinsic effect on panic disorder. There are some studies that suggest that sleeplessness may lead to increased vulnerability to colds and other minor infections, but these are minor infections only; and the effect is minor. There are certain diseases that do indeed get worse with lack of sleep, among them schizophrenia, but none are <u>caused</u> by lack of sleep. The central importance of getting a good night's sleep, like the importance of eating 3 meals a day, or the importance of having a good bowel movement, is a myth.

But insomnia is unpleasant and exasperating; and it can become a habit. Ideally, one would like to be able to convince an insomniac that going without sleep for a couple of nights is trivial and not worth worrying about. The insomnia, then, would very likely disappear. But these habits of mind are so ingrained, merely lecturing to such a person will not work. Also unlikely to be successful are attempts to get him or her to stay up purposely for a couple of days just to prove that nothing bad will come of it! But less severe treatments have proven successful. The following is a treatment program that works if the health worrier can be persuaded to follow its rules.

<u>Treatment program for insomnia</u>

1. Simply lying down in bed should produce a feeling of sleepiness and will do so if lying in bed is associated exclusively with sleeping. Someone who is in bed off and on all day will not get sleepy going to bed. That means, eating or watching television in bed is not permitted. No reading in bed is allowed unless a few minutes of reading is part of a bedtime ritual. Patients are resistant to this advice. They <u>like</u> lying around in bed, relaxing. It is hard to convince them that insomnia, and their other symptoms too, are tied

up inextricably with accustomed patterns of behavior. But it is so. The reason why the sleep patterns of hospital patients get fouled up is that they stay in bed all day long. Reclining in a chair next to the bed is okay.

2. It does not matter when insomniacs go to bed; but they should get out of bed at the same time every morning 7 days a week. That means they should get up on Sunday morning at the same time they would if they were going to work, <u>even if they have slept poorly all the previous week.</u> The temptation to "catch up" on missed sleep is very strong; but if they sleep late on Sunday, or any other day, they will not fall asleep promptly that night. If they get up at the same time every day and <u>avoid naps</u> they will sooner or later-usually within a matter of days - start falling asleep at an appropriate time. But, of course, they have to put up with being sleepy, purposely, for a while, which is unpleasant.

3. Insomniacs should not look at a clock during the night. It should be turned to the wall. Discovering that it is 2: 1 0 and then 2:20 and the 2:30 A.M. is upsetting and serves no useful purpose. It is a reminder of how much sleep is being missed, and, consequently, causes people to become more anxious and, therefore, wakeful. Besides, unbelievable though it may seem, they are usually asleep between 2:10 and 2:20 A.M. and between 2:20 and 2:30 A.M. Insomniacs always sleep more than they realize.

As in so many other areas, psychotherapy is directed at helping patients determine the truth of matters. This usually means getting them to distrust their convictions, their perceptions, and their memories. It is uphill work. I sent one woman who claimed she was entirely sleepless day after day to a sleep clinic. She woke up the following morning announcing, "See, I told you, I don't sleep at all," when we had an EEG record documenting that she had been asleep the whole night! I cannot understand why most patients resist turning the clock to the wall. Looking at it in the middle of the night gives no satisfaction, but they do.

4. Probably no one should use the snooze alarm. At best, someone is awakened from deep sleep only to return to a lighter, less critical stage of sleep. Insomniacs, who are already complaining of insufficient sleep, thereby get less. More significantly, however, someone who presses the snooze alarm repeatedly has no clear cue as to when to get out of bed. Ordinarily-properly- someone hears the alarm ring, perhaps from across the room, and gets up to turn it off. The alarm is a signal to wake up. Someone who uses the snooze alarm, not infrequently 4 or 5 times on a single morning, has no clear signal to wake up once and for all. Each time the alarm rings, he, or she, has to decide whether this time is the time finally to get up. Or not. The alarm should be set for the last possible moment and when it rings, the sleeper should get out of bed.

5. People who have trouble falling asleep should not drink regular coffee after 3 P.M.; and those who wake up during the night should not drink alcohol after dinnertime. The alcohol is sedating at first, but activating a few hours later when it wears off.

6. Finally, no one should take sleeping medications more than three nights in a row. Tolerance develops quickly. Also, these drugs may cause sleepiness in the morning. No sleeping pill works noticeably better than the others.

There are other causes of poor sleep, such as sleep apnea, which causes inadequate breathing, thereby disrupting the normal sleep architecture. Still other, more unusual, conditions may also cause insomnia. The treatment for insomnia sketched out above usually works. If it does not, a referral to a specialized sleep clinic is indicated.

Bad Ideas about Medication

Health worriers tend to believe:

1. That all medicines are inherently dangerous and should be avoided if possible.

2. That they, themselves, are particularly sensitive to, and likely to, have a bad reaction to a variety of medicines.
3. That smaller doses of medicine are always safer than large doses.
4. That "natural" products such as "herbs," discussed in more detail in <u>Worried Sick? The Workbook,</u> are safer than pharmacological agents produced by the large drug companies.
5. That there is a conspiracy among the larger drug companies - perhaps in an alliance with other parts of the medical establishment - to foist expensive drugs on the public rather than cheaper "natural" substances.
6. That these drug companies are likely to release medicines to the public without first properly testing their safety, even if doing so puts them at risk of billion dollar lawsuits.

They have similar Bad Ideas about other medical interventions such as x-ray studies, anesthesia and surgical operations.

As a consequence of these views, health worriers may go without the benefits of modern medicine. They are resistant to taking medicines that could be helpful to them- particularly when those medicines are psychoactive, such as the anti-depressants. Not uncommonly, they hesitate to take antibiotics, cardiac drugs, pain relievers and hormones. Although none of these agents are entirely safe under all circumstances, their advantages are unmistakable.

These Bad Ideas, like the other Bad Ideas mentioned throughout this book are false; and they lead to trouble. <u>Refusal to take drugs that are indicated can cause worsening of illness with the result that more medical intervention becomes necessary;</u> and sometimes death is the result.

Health worriers derive Bad Ideas not only from articles in the popular press - of which there are many - but, as usual, from their own personal experiences. In order to understand why, it is necessary to discuss the placebo response.

<u>The Placebo Response</u>

Doctors sometimes give drugs that they know have no intrinsic value because they have long recognized that the act of giving the drug itself has beneficial effects. These are called placebos. Throughout most of recorded history the <u>only</u> drugs available were placebos. A typical situation in which such a drug might be prescribed nowadays is in the treatment of pain in a context in which real pain medication might complicate other treatments which the patient is undergoing at the same time. Sometimes the physician is concerned that the patient is becoming addicted to morphine or to other such potent medications and wishes to lessen their use by giving a placebo instead. One example of the use of placebos was the former practice of treating anxious patients with biweekly injections of vitamin B 12, despite it being well-known at that time that the only legitimate use of B 12 was to prevent pernicious anemia. In those years there was not a widespread availability of real tranquilizers. I like to think that the physicians' charging five dollars for an injection that cost them 15 cents was not a relevant consideration. Some of the minor tranquilizers that are among the most commonly prescribed drugs in the world today have so little effect in the doses in which they are often given that they too might be considered placebos. Many over-the-counter drugs are placebos, including some sleeping medications. <u>Placebos work because the patient's expectations alone tend to produce the desired results.</u> When the drug is recommended by a respected or charismatic physician, they are very likely to work - <u>not just on suggestible persons, but on everyone</u>. In desperate situations, for example, when the patient's life is threatened, they may work dramatically.

What is not widely appreciated, however, is that <u>placebos can have side-effects!</u> Once again, the reason is that the results of taking a drug can be influenced strongly by the patient's expectations. The following list of side-effects is taken from the placebo arm of a study on anti-depressants. These are patients who were given dummy pills that resembled the real medication. Neither they nor the physician knew whether they were taking the real medication or the placebo.

Under these circumstances those patients who took the placebo complained of the following symptoms:

19% of such patients complained of:		Headache
7%	"	Dizziness
3%	"	Tremor
12%	"	Nausea
9%	"	Diarrhea
6%	"	Constipation
2%	"	Abdominal pain
8%	"	Fatigue
9%	"	Insomnia
6%	"	Somnolence
4%	"	Agitation
2%	"	Male sexual dysfunction
2%	"	Abnormal vision

It should be noted that many of these symptoms are those often associated with stress; but by no means do these exhaust the side-effects placebos cause. In this particular study 42 kinds of symptoms were common enough to list by percentage. Many others occur rarely. Probably no subjective symptom is so unusual it cannot be produced by a placebo given under the right circumstances. This particular study is in no way unusual, although the proportions of the various side-effects will vary depending on what drug the patients think they may be receiving.

There are many persons, including the majority of health worriers, who expect to develop side effects when they take drugs; and consequently they do. Even from placebos. This effect is well - recognized and complicates the management of medical illness. Someone who invariably develops side-effects comes naturally to believe that he, or she, is peculiarly vulnerable; and believing that makes it so! That idea is sustained also by those psychological factors mentioned in Chapter II, i.e. selective attention, selective memory, and so on. The cure is the same for all Bad Ideas: more information. The trick, as usual, is to engage the patient in those cognitive exercises which allow new information to become integrated into the patient's point of view. An additional strategy for doctors concerned about limiting a drug's side effects is described below.

First, of course, the doctor should present a detailed, honest account of the benefits of a particular drug, and also of the <u>most likely</u> side-effects. The patient's questions should be answered even if they seem obsessional or irrational.

Second, any measure that encourages the patient to <u>try</u> the drug is helpful. Usually, the first pill is the hardest to take. The patient should understand that side-effects of drugs, when they do occur, usually disappear promptly upon stopping the drug, so their fear of side-effects is not a reason not to give the drug a try. Sometimes I take the drug along with the patient for the first few days. Not all drugs. I know most drugs are safe and produce no significant side-effects; but some do. A few days is usually long enough for placebo effects to wear off.

Third, because placebo effects occur immediately and wear off usually in only a few days, the patient suffering with a side-effect should be encouraged by the doctor to stay on the drug for a little while to see if the side-effect fades. The doctor should not be in a rush to switch to another drug unless the side-effect is inherently dangerous, such as an asthma attack, or of a kind not likely to be psychological in origin, such as a rash. Changing drugs immediately sustains the patient's Bad Ideas about medication.

If a doctor takes enough time to do these things, most patients can overcome their prejudices and participate sensibly in their own medical care.

Chapter Eleven: Common Clinical Errors

Somewhere along the way of life, for reasons described in previous chapters, health worriers have developed a prejudice - really a series of prejudices - about their health. These sum to a kind of uh-oh point of view, an expectation that at any moment their bodies can break down catastrophically. They do not usually worry about common illnesses which they know from their own experience are usually transient and insignificant. They are unlikely to worry about a cold, unless they can somehow imagine it turning into pneumonia. And even pneumonia is not likely to frighten them very much. They worry about illnesses that have the potential to devastate their lives. Since they are not usually seriously ill with any obvious symptoms of such an illness, they look for subtle evidence of these conditions in order to catch them in time and cure them if possible. Some such illnesses can develop, they know, with no signs or symptoms at all, so they are in the habit of worrying even when they are entirely well. As suggested in the last few chapters, their worries about getting sick can be varied and idiosyncratic; but, obviously, the diseases they worry about most are those that are known to be the most serious. Some of them are crippling. Most of them are fatal, potentially, at least. There are not a great many diseases that lurk quietly without significant signs or symptoms and at the same time are likely to be fatal. So, these particular illnesses appear over and over again in the preoccupations of different health worriers. They may switch from worrying about one illness over a period of time to worrying about another; but it is usually just one of these that is the focus of their concerns. The particular illness that frightens them the most is determined by chance factors: did some member of the family or even a friend die of that condition; has that particular illness received a lot of publicity recently; did a doctor mention that condition in passing; and so on. Usually the patient's symptoms, such as they are, have little to do with the illness the patient is worried about currently, although he or she may think otherwise.

Another error they make is universal: <u>Invariably, health worriers think the particular illness they dread is more common than it really is</u>. An illness such as breast cancer, for example, may have a lifetime incidence of one in eight women, a well-known statistic; but the chance of a woman in her thirties, forties, or fifties, developing the condition is very much lower. The chance of the cancer proving fatal is still less. Also, there is a natural tendency for people to over-estimate the prevalence of a disease they have run into personally. Put a different way, they underestimate the extent of statistical variation. Because three children in the neighborhood have developed leukemia, it does not mean it is a common disease. Still less does it mean there is something in the neighborhood such as pollution that is causing the disease. In general, health worriers need to be reminded that people get sick over and over again over the course of a lifetime, but are not likely to get more than one fatal illness.

These factors and others tend to lead health worriers into the same mistakes. Certain common medical conditions are routinely confused with others that are more serious and much less common. People end up worrying about the wrong disease. Some of the more typical worries are described below. Each example could be multiplied many times over.

Palpitations and/or Heart Disease

Elizabeth was a 34-year old woman who described herself as "capable, but always worried about something or other." From time to time she worried about her health. Recently, however, a particular health worry had preoccupied her entirely so that she found it difficult to manage her day to day household routine. She had begun to think she was about to have a heart attack.

The problem had started a few weeks before when she was lying quietly in bed watching television. Suddenly, she noticed a fluttery feeling in the middle of her chest. A few moments later the feeling came again. She sat up abruptly, frightened by the thought that her heart was beating abnormally. She pressed her finger hard against her breastbone, feeling vaguely for her heartbeat and trying, perhaps, to make it come right. But a few seconds later - or a few minutes later, she could not tell - the feeling returned again, lasting this time a little longer. She shook her husband and asked him to hold her hand, or take her pulse, or just wake up and talk to her for a few minutes. She explained anxiously that her heart had begun sputtering, that it was skipping a beat. There and there again. And now it was going a mile a minute. She thought she was going to die, she told him. Her husband listened patiently for a few minutes, offered a few words of encouragement, then rolled over and went back to sleep. Elizabeth got out of bed and paced about, trying to calm herself down. Her chest hurt now when she pressed a knuckle against it. Was that a sign of a heart attack? She knew that pain was a sign of a heart attack. After about an hour or so she calmed down. The fluttery feeling seemed to have gone away; and she went to sleep.

The next night something similar happened. This time she was reading when the fluttery feeling recurred and then came again every few minutes interspersed with a new feeling, a sudden thump in the middle of her chest. She roused her husband, who was sleeping again, and prevailed on him to drive her to the emergency room of a nearby hospital. Despite her protesting that there might be something wrong with her heart, the nursing staff put her into a room where she waited for three hours before being seen by a physician and where her husband once again went to sleep. Finally she was given an EKG, which was read as normal. The emergency room doctor told her he could find nothing wrong with her heart, then told her, for some unexplained reason, that she should see her own doctor in the morning, gave her a tranquilizer, and sent her home. She had trouble sleeping the remainder of the night because she felt her pulse in her neck when she lay on her left side; and she kept waiting for her heart to skip a beat.

The next day her doctor took another EKG and told her that her heart was beating normally "except for a couple of premature heart contractions." It was probably PVCs, as these beats were called, that were causing the funny feelings in her chest.

"Not to worry," he said

"But, what causes these things?" she asked.

"It's not really abnormal," he replied.

"Not really? Well, suppose...I mean, I never had them before".

"You probably had them before. You just didn't notice them."

"Forget it. If anything like this had happened to me before, I would have noticed it."

"Well, there's no reason to worry about it."

"Suppose it gets worse..."

This colloquy went on long enough for the doctor to decide to order a Holter monitor. This is a device a patient wears all day long in order to monitor heart function continuously. When the results of the test were reported back, another conversation ensued.

Doctor: Well, as I expected, you had a number of PVCs during the day, but nothing to worry about.

Elizabeth: But that day I didn't have so many. I could tell. It wasn't as bad as it usually is. These symptoms are like the police; they're never around when you want them.

Doctor: It doesn't matter. You're okay. Don't worry.

But Elizabeth did worry. She consulted a cardiologist who told her in almost the same words what her family doctor had said to her. But she was still not consoled. She could not believe that these PVCs, whatever they were, might not suddenly accelerate - maybe if she was under stress - and get worse and worse and just possibly cause a heart attack. Seeing that her anxiety could not be relieved, the cardiologist suggested that she could, if she wished, take one of two kinds of drugs, or both. The first, of course, was a tranquilizer to calm her down. The second was a beta blocker which would diminish the number of PVCs and slow her heart rate, even if she got excited. But he emphasized, she did not need to take either drug if she chose not to.

For the next number of months, Elizabeth agonized about whether or not to take these drugs. On one hand she was still afraid of what she now began to think of as her "heart condition". On the other hand, like most health worriers, she was afraid of the medication. She ended up taking the drugs intermittently, even randomly, and in sub-clinical doses, too low to have any effect at all. Although not as desperate as she was when she first visited her doctor, she continued to worry.

Good things to know

If Elizabeth understood, or could have been led to understand, certain facts she would have worried less.

1. Premature ventricular contractions, PVCs, were, indeed, likely to be the cause of her symptoms. They usually cause fluttery feelings or an occasional thump in the chest, exactly as she experienced them.

2. Dangerous heart arrhythmias, for there are such, present differently and look different on the Holter monitor.

3. PVCs often occur at a rate of more than five an hour in totally normal people. And a number of otherwise normal people get many more.

4. Those who get many PVCs have been followed for many years with no increased incidence of heart disease.

5. Everyone who gets upset will have an elevated heart rate. This is normal and can go on for long periods of time without damaging the heart. The heart cannot beat faster than a certain rate depending on the person's age and physical condition. It cannot be driven past that point by stress or exercise; and it is not damaged by going as fast as it can - any more than running a faucet wide open can damage the plumbing.

6. The term "heart attack" usually refers to a myocardial infarction, the sudden blocking of coronary arteries that have already been

damaged by certain diseases such as atherosclerosis. <u>Heart attacks are rare in women of Elizabeth's age.</u>

7. Unimportant though they may be, PVCs can be diminished in number by an exercise program.

One might ask, why cannot the health worrier simply accept the doctor's reassurance without going into all this detail. First of all, it must be acknowledged that they cannot, for reasons outlined in the previous chapters. They have preconceptions about their own health and about other things that outweigh and overshadow anything a doctor may tell them. <u>Nevertheless, they can learn not to worry about a particular medical condition by learning the relevant medical facts.</u> Instead of taking the doctor's word, they can see for themselves. But with no training in medicine can they obtain the information they need? Yes. The resources they can use — beyond their doctor's advice — to learn about whatever condition they may have include magazine articles, the internet, medical textbooks and journal articles. But some things must be kept in mind:

1. Magazines are written to be entertaining or exciting. Therefore, the account they give of anything at all is likely to be overly dramatic. That means full of the unusual and the calamitous. Doctors are not quoted accurately; and often facts are distorted. Still, these articles are better read than skipped over. At least they provide some information. The bad things one can imagine on one's own always go beyond those things likely to happen; so avoiding listening to, or reading about, an account of a dreaded disease makes matters worse.

2. The internet makes available some very reliable information, but also some not so reliable. Some web sites are run by professionals; others are not. <u>Those web sites that are run by groups of individuals affected by a particular illness are likely, it should be kept in mind, to represent the views of those worst affected by that condition.</u> Those who have recovered are no longer likely to participate.

3. Medical textbooks have a lot of specialized jargon which seems indecipherable at first but which is plain enough with a medical dictionary. <u>Since they are written for medical students, however, they include all the possible consequences of an illness, not just those that are most likely</u>. Also, they do not always indicate the sequence in which symptoms develop. Sometimes health worriers put their particular symptoms together with a particular (usually devastating) disease without taking into account the fact that if they had that disease, they would have first developed a whole bunch of other symptoms. For example, AIDS may sometimes be the cause of urinary infections, but it would be very unusual for that to happen as the first symptom of AIDS. Put differently, developing a urinary infection should not cause someone to worry about AIDS.

There is a fourth source of information of interest to health worriers and, as in the case of the others, a source also of concern and misunderstanding — that is, the drug insert. This is a page or so of detailed information packaged in every drug bottle. It is intended for the prescribing physician and includes a description of mode of action of the drug, method of dispensing, and side effects along with other facts such as how the drug is metabolized and removed from the body. Identical information appears in the Physician's Desk Reference (the PDR). A naïve person glancing though these pages would never want to take any medication since the listed side effects are so many. If someone taking five medicines at the same time suffered some sort of medical mishap, that problem might very well be reported as a potential complication of all of these drugs, even though only one might have been at fault, or none. Because someone develops a rash, for instance, following the start of a new medicine, it does not mean the rash was due to the medicine. Rashes occur randomly in some people. They also show up in certain viral syndromes a few days after other symptoms have developed and after some particular medicine has been started. In this case the medicine is likely to be blamed for the rash. For reasons mentioned previously, some wary people are likely to develop certain particular kinds of reactions to any drugs. These are the physical manifestations of anxiety.

In order to judge the real side effects of a drug, the list of side effects should be compared against the corresponding effects of a placebo. These are often listed in the PDR. If 15% of those people who took a drug reported that they got a headache and a similar percentage of those who took a matching placebo also got a headache, it is reasonable to presume that the drug does not cause headaches. As usual, the patient should not be interested in the very worst complication of a drug, which is not infrequently death, but in which side effects are likely. Of course, the prescribing physician should have already mentioned these.

A good use of the drug inserts or the PDR is to check drug interactions. It would be nice to think that every physician checks to see if a new drug interacts with drugs the patient is already on; but unfortunately, that is not always the case And as there are more and more drugs, there are more and more drug interactions. For example, those drugs that are used to slow blood clotting are affected by 20 or more other drugs, some of which may have one effect and at the same time to a different degree the opposite effect! Although it is not unreasonable for patients to find out as much as possible about drugs prescribed for their benefit, no one should think that by reading these pages he or she can become a better judge of the appropriateness of a medication than his or her doctor.

The facts that Elizabeth, or any other health worrier, would find useful fall into two main categories: facts about the patient's symptoms or illness, as the doctor has defined it, and facts about the more serious illness which springs so readily to the mind of the patient. Put differently, health worriers need to learn more about their real illness and also about the illness that haunts their nightmare fantasies. After an initial period of heightened anxiety, learning more about each will make the real illness seem more and more likely and the dreaded illness less and less.

Chest Pain and/or Heart Disease

Peter, like Elizabeth, worried that he might have heart disease, but for a different reason. He had begun worrying when he was a child and was witness to his uncle dying of a heart attack. His father too had a heart attack at an early age. Peter, who was inclined in general to think of himself as unlucky, became convinced that he was going to die of a heart attack before he was fifty. Having passed this magic age, he began to worry more rather than less since he was now living on borrowed time. These background anxieties worsened abruptly one evening when he was required to speak at a business dinner. As soon as he finished eating, he began to experience a midline chest pain that seemed to radiate into his left arm. The pain worsened when he had an alcoholic drink to help him calm down. After a few minutes it receded completely only to return a little while later when he found himself rushing to make the last train home. He felt better, though, as soon as he got on the train. That night the pain returned forcibly as soon as he lay down but improved somewhat when he turned onto his left side or sat up. Finally, after pacing half the night he became convinced he was having a heart attack. His wife drove him to the emergency room of a hospital where he was admitted overnight and certain blood tests were done. He was told after an EKG that he had "tachycardia" but no evidence of a heart attack. That pronouncement seemed too vague to him to be reassuring; but following discharge the next morning he went to work trying to put the pain out of mind.

Over the next week he found himself "testing" the pain, which worsened, he noticed, upon bending over. His chest was tender too, especially over the left side. Often the pain went away quickly only to return again in the middle of the night. He put off visiting his doctor because he was convinced the doctor would tell him to give up drinking alcohol and eating steak, which was his favorite food - and very likely, also, give up smoking. Also, he was pretty sure the doctor would scold him again as he had many times before about his weight. 280 pounds, the doctor insisted, was too much for someone with a family history of heart disease.

When the doctor was finally consulted, he ordered a number of tests after which he made a diagnosis of gastroesophageal reflux disorder (GERD) and not any kind of heart disease. Peter went along with the treatment program recommended by the doctor, which did, indeed, involve certain dietary changes and certainly smoking cessation; but he maintained to members of his family that his pain was typical of heart disease. Therefore, he insisted that one of these days it was likely to worsen; and he was going to drop dead. Even the doctor thought he might die someday of heart disease, he went on to say.

Good Things to Know:

1. Peter was right in thinking that his chest pain was consistent with the possibility of a heart attack, but he would have felt better if he knew that similar pain could be produced by GERD, including radiation of the pain into the left arm. The reason is simple: the same nerve supplies the heart and the esophagus and sends roots into the left arm and to a number of other places too.

2. Although the distinction between the two conditions cannot be made on the basis of the pain alone, it is nevertheless true that the pains they cause are in their most characteristic form different one from the other as follows:

GERD pain is worsened by dietary excesses such as a big, spicy or fat laden meal and alcohol ingestion. It is worsened by lying down and relieved by sitting up or standing. It tends to recur at intervals, particularly at night, and recede the rest of the time. It is usually relieved promptly by antacids.

The pain of a heart attack can vary from crushing to nonexistent; but typically it is a severe, constricting pain that can come on at any time, is prolonged, and relieved only by powerful analgesics. It is not altered by movement or made worse by pressing on the chest. Although Peter's pain could have been caused by a heart attack, it was more suggestive of GERD. And had he read about both conditions, he would have found reasons to worry less. The pain of coronary artery disease, angina, can also be confused with a heart attack; but it too, has a characteristic appearance. It too may occur at any time but is likely to appear especially during exercise or at times of emotional stress. It lasts only a matter of minutes.

3. The heart attack, which Peter thought was inevitable, can more and more often be prevented and, like GERD, can be treated. The rate of death from heart disease has fallen steadily over the last 50 years, even though it still kills more people than any other disease. Having a family history of premature heart disease is a risk factor, but not a sentence of doom. To an extent the familial risk is mediated through high cholesterol, which can be controlled by diet and drugs. Other risk factors such as hypertension and diabetes can also be treated successfully. With determination and the help of various medications, even inveterate cigarette smokers can stop. And even small amounts of exercise further lower the risk of a heart attack. If Peter had understood the risks better and the measures he could take to ameliorate the risks, he would have been less pessimistic. Some measures such as weight loss and stopping cigarette smoking would lessen the risk of a heart attack and improve his GERD at the same time.

Whenever anyone is worried about anything, actively confronting the problem will not only lessen whatever damage may be associated with it but will also have a good effect on morale. Doing something makes people feel better. Peter plainly had a lot he could do.

Headaches and/or a Brain Tumor

Norman had always worried about brain tumors. Consequently, when a friend of his who was a medical student told him he was about to attend a lecture on brain tumors, Norman invited himself along. Although the lecture dealt optimistically with treatments that had recently been developed, the lecturer also opined that "brain tumors are no damn good;" and that phrase was all that Norman remembered.

Over the next 20 years Norman became unusually successful. He managed a family business, sold it, and invested the money in a still larger business of which he became the president in due course. He married happily and fathered three children. He was well regarded by everyone. In particular, his business acumen was thought to be only one aspect of a larger intelligence: he had common sense. But on the single matter of his health, he seemed irrational. He worried about various conditions at various times, but he was preoccupied especially with the possibility of his having a brain tumor. The symptoms that set him to worrying were not always the same.

One summer when Norman was 21, his hay fever seemed to be worse than usual. In addition to a runny nose and red eyes he developed a persistent pain over his right cheek and the right side of his forehead. The whole area around his right eye was tender and swollen a little. He began to run a low grade fever. Then his nose began to bleed. After he was examined, he asked his doctor:

"Can a brain tumor cause a steady pain in the eye day after day?"

"Well, yes," replied the doctor, "but what you've got is an acute sinusitis."

Good Things to Know:

An allergic rhinitis, which is common and which causes a runny nose, can become infected and lead to a sinusitis. This infection causes a steady pain over the affected sinuses, above an eye or below it, although sometimes the pain can be referred to a different part of the head altogether. It can develop quickly and can indeed include some bleeding from the nose.

Brain tumor headaches, on the other hand, do not usually

cause redness of the eyes, a runny nose and pain over the sinuses. There is no tenderness; and the pain does not usually become apparent suddenly and very severely. Brain tumors do not cause fever. And, of course, sinusitis is very common and brain tumors are not.

Only a few months later Norman developed aching pain in his upper jaw directly below the area that had hurt him previously. If he bit down hard on something, or ate ice cream, the pain became stabbing. His first thought, as usual, was of a brain tumor. This time, however, he already knew enough to suspect a different cause of his pain, at least enough to visit a dentist before going for further consultation. Following a root canal excision performed by an endodontist, he felt entirely well.

During the next few years he remained well except for occasional diffuse headaches which were readily alleviated by over-the-counter medicines. Perhaps because he had had similar headaches as long as he could remember, all of which had gone away in time, he never worried about them. But one summer he found himself waking up every Sunday morning with a throbbing headache, usually only on one side of the head, although not always on the same side. The headaches were largely unrelieved by aspirin but went away usually during the course of the day, leaving a strange tenderness of his scalp for a few days. Naturally, he wondered about a brain tumor; but because he was on vacation, he did not immediately go to a doctor.

When he returned home, however, a much more dramatic headache frightened him. He was sitting quietly in a movie theater, feeling fine, when suddenly he realized he could not see one side of the screen. He had gone blind! Superimposed over Harrison Ford's face was a line of bright lights that danced before his eyes. They went on sparkling even when his eyes were closed. Over the course of a few minutes they got bigger and moved off to one side, thankfully restoring his vision. But 20 minutes later, on the other side of his head, a pounding headache began. The pain was so extreme he thought this time it had to be a brain tumor. Whether from the pain itself or from being upset, he began to feel sick to his stomach.

"Doc, can a brain tumor cause really bad headaches?" he asked the neurologist whom he had gone to see the next day "and bright lights in your vision?"

"Yes," the doctor said.

"What about feeling nauseous?"

"Sure, but what you've got is migraine."

Good Things to Know:

Migraine is a vascular headache, which is why it throbs. Like many other conditions it is both physical and psychological in nature. The headaches can be brought on in a genetically vulnerable individual by alcohol, certain foods, sleeping too much and by stress, or, more usually, by relaxing after a period of stress. It can be very painful and can also cause sensitivity to light and nausea, even vomiting.

Common migraine, or "weekend headache," is, indeed common, perhaps the most common kind of headache. Classical migraine, which may occur in the same individual, has a very characteristic presentation, exactly as Norman experienced it. Brain tumors do not cause this precise sequence of physical symptoms. Brain tumors do not appear on one side of the head one time and on the other side a week later. Very severe, throbbing headaches are more typical of migraines than a brain tumor.

It would not be reasonable to expect that Norman, or any other health worrier, would know all this as part of a fund of general information. Even someone who did would likely be frightened by going partially blind, even temporarily. But like most health worriers, Norman continued to worry even after being reassured by his doctor. At that point reading about these conditions on his own would have made a difference.

But there were more problems to come. A number of years later Norman may or may not have injured himself on a camping trip with his son. That is, he went to sleep one night in his sleeping bag and woke up the next morning with a stiff neck. A few days later he began to have a new kind of headache. The pain may, or may not, have been located in part where his stiff neck had hurt him; but the principal pain he had extended around his head like a tight band. Unlike his migraine headaches, which he had not had for over a year, this pain was dull and steady and worse in the evening. The pain went away with aspirin only to return the next day and the day after. By now Norman was hesitant to rush to a doctor since he felt embarrassed. But he still feared the worst. Over the next month he had an unchanging headache every day for a week followed by a week of no headaches and again headaches the following week.

Norman returned finally to the same neurologist and as before had a number of questions, more about brain tumors than about the likely cause of his particular symptoms.

"Can a brain tumor cause daily headaches?"

"It usually does."

"Well, my headaches aren't very painful. Is that possible with a brain tumor?"

"It is possible."

"Well," said Norman nervously, "my headaches get better with aspirin. That couldn't happen with a brain tumor, could it?"

"Well, it could. But what I think you have is a tension headache."

"But, could it possibly be a brain tumor?"

"Anything is possible."

The neurologist chose on this occasion to order a CAT scan, which ruled out a brain tumor.

Good Things to Know:

First of all, it is good to know that CAT scans <u>can</u> rule out a brain tumor. Health worriers can stop worrying at that point, at least until the next time.

Norman might have worried less waiting for the results of the CAT scan if he had known that tension headaches present typically as a tight band across the forehead. Brain tumors typically do not. Tension headaches may persist for very long periods of time; but they are usually intermittent. Brain tumor headaches do not usually skip an entire week. Also, brain tumors often cause other symptoms besides headaches. Norman had no unusual sensations, no loss of muscular function, no convulsions, and no deficit of any of the special senses. As the neurologist had informed him, his physical examination was normal. He had no weakness, alteration in balance or abnormal reflexes. He had no abnormal changes in his eye grounds that might have suggested an increase in intracranial pressure. Did the lack of these other symptoms and signs mean that there was no chance at all of a brain tumor? No. This sort of question, the kind that occurred naturally to Norman, is designed to elicit the wrong answer. The right question is: what condition am I likely to have? Not: what is the worst conceivable condition I can have? The neurologist's response, "anything is possible," is always true. For example, it probably cannot be said of any head pain that it cannot be caused by or be associated with a brain tumor. In the same sense one could say there is a risk inherent in walking down a street since automobiles can, and every once in a while do, jump the curb and run down pedestrians. But should this possibility spring to mind every time one takes a stroll?

On the subject of headaches and brain tumors, a good rule of thumb is this: any new headache that persists for a number of weeks should be evaluated.

A 26 year old man had been in psychotherapy for a number of years for a range of neurotic complaints including conflicts at work, with his friends, and in the sexual sphere. He also had a long history of bizarre somatic complaints including shooting pains and tingling sensations, which lasted only long enough to be replaced by the next physical symptom. Acknowledging all of this, he referred to himself dispassionately as a "head case."

There came a time when he developed a new symptom: each

afternoon when he lay down to take a nap, a pain "zinged" around his head. The pain was relieved promptly by opening a window and taking a deep breath of fresh air. This strange headache did not seem very different from any of the other evanescent aches and pains that he always complained about. The treating psychiatrist also took into consideration the fact that brain tumors have a bimodal distribution; that is, they occur most frequently in children and in the elderly. This young man was in- between. Nevertheless, when the headache persisted unchanging for almost a month, the psychiatrist referred him for neurological examination. He was found to have a pituitary tumor that was readily cured surgically. When he recovered, he continued to have conflicts in all the various aspects of his life, but the headaches were gone.

Diarrhea and/or Rectal Bleeding and/or Colon Cancer

Just as Norman had one physical problem after another that suggested to him the possibility of a brain tumor, Arlene had a number of symptoms that kept her worrying about another potentially fatal disease: colon cancer. Once again there was a family history of this disease. Often it is just such an accident of fortune that causes the health worrier to obsess about one particular illness instead of any of a number of others, some of which are more likely. In the case of both heart disease and colon cancer, there is a true familial risk; but for many other persons, the particular illness of concern does not run in families and may not even have occurred in a family member. A neighbor dying dramatically of that illness is enough.

Given the fact that her mother and aunt had developed colon cancer - although at an advanced age - it was understandable that Arlene would think that she too might get it. In fact, she had complained of "stomach problems" dating back to early adolescence when she experienced abdominal cramps that lasted off and on for months. Her doctor at that time considered Crohn's disease, which is one form of inflammatory bowel disease, but put off x-ray studies and further diagnostic procedures since she did not have diarrhea, which is another feature of the illness. In time the cramps went away.

When she was older and living away from home at college, she developed what was diagnosed at the time as irritable bowel syndrome, I.B.S., a condition that then persisted more or less throughout her life. Her symptoms included, once again, lower abdominal cramps relieved this time by multiple bowel movements every morning. Her cramps were worse, particularly on days when she was studying for examinations or otherwise under stress. Occasionally, perversely, she became constipated, especially after using the antispasmodic drugs which were prescribed to control her diarrhea. During her junior year, following a vacation in Puerto Rico, her diarrhea worsened significantly and it was thought by her physician that she might have become infected by parasites. The medical work up she underwent took place over a period of weeks and included:

First, a purged specimen of stool. An examination was made on fresh diarrhea brought on by ingesting citrate of magnesia, a substance so profoundly distasteful it caused her to throw up the first time she took it. This test was performed to search for ova and parasites and was reported back negative.

She was sent, then, for a barium enema with contrast studies. This involved instilling barium and air into her rectum, which was corked, briefly – with a cork! The study too was read as normal.

Finally, she was sigmoidoscoped. This test allowed the gastroenterologist to visualize directly the mucosa in the rectum. Finding normal mucosa, as he did, made ulcerative colitis, another inflammatory bowel disease, unlikely. Colon cancer, which the gastroenterologist explained to Arlene was very unlikely at her age, was also "largely ruled out." This response seemed not entirely definite to Arlene who had begun her lifelong preoccupation with colon cancer. When she pressed him repeatedly to be more exact about the risk of cancer and a number of other diseases, he informed her, perhaps tongue in cheek, as follows:

218

Colon cancer was 98% ruled out.

Ulcerative colitis was 96% ruled out.

Parasites were 98.5% ruled out.

But Crohn's disease, he owned, was only partially ruled out. Still, since her diarrhea was free of blood, he was not prepared to perform further diagnostic tests at that time. He also mentioned in passing that, of course, other conditions also caused diarrhea. This casual remark provoked another 15 minutes of conversation, which left Arlene more worried rather than less. The doctor ended by telling Arlene that he had been "97% sure" she had only irritable bowel syndrome even before ordering all these tests. He recommended higher doses of the antispasmodic drugs she had been taking all along. It was not long before her symptoms subsided. Nevertheless, she worried still that she might have colon cancer farther up the colon than the sigmoidoscope could reach. It was during this period that her aunt died of colon cancer.

A few years later, now in graduate school, Arlene noticed some blood on her toilet paper! Since she had been asked repeatedly previously about the presence of blood in her stool, she took this as a sign of the cancer that she had so long been anticipating. After an emergency consultation that evening her doctor told her she had hemorrhoids and that they did not require treatment. This simple explanation of rectal bleeding did not entirely assuage her concerns since her doctor when pressed also told her there was no way he could be certain she did not have a colon cancer in addition to hemorrhoids.

Over the next few days her abdominal cramps worsened. Her gastroenterologist, motivated mostly by the desire to reassure Arlene once and for all that she was not suffering from any serious disease, ordered a barium swallow to rule out Crohn's disease of the small intestine and then performed a colonoscopy to visualize the entire colon.

"I am 110% sure you don't have colon cancer," he informed

her subsequently, opting to sound a little more definite than is the custom of most physicians.

And Arlene did, indeed, feel relieved. However, when her rectal bleeding, which waxed and waned, waxed more than usual six months later, she returned to her doctor to inquire anxiously whether she might now have colon cancer.

Good Things to Know:

1. Arlene would have worried less if she understood how very uncommon colon cancer was at her age, even in individuals with a family history of the disease.

2. She would have become less upset when her cramps were severe if she had known that cramps are not an initial presentation of colon cancer.

3. She would have been less worried if she had understood that bright red blood visible on toilet paper was likely to come from anal lesions such as hemorrhoids or other problems easily accessible to and diagnosed by rectal examination.

4. Colon cancer is thought to evolve over a period of years, going through precancerous stages such as polyps that are readily treatable. A careful colonoscopy that showed no evidence of disease means that symptoms developing a year or two later would not be due to cancer.

5. Irritable bowel syndrome does not lead to colon cancer.

6. Colon cancer when it does occur is readily curable in its early stages. Therefore, a proper program of surveillance instituted at the proper age should make it very unlikely that even a vulnerable person such as Arlene should die of this disease.

Arlene's case demonstrates the general rule that health worriers are likely to undergo more medical testing and procedures than the ordinary person who comes to the same doctor with the same physical complaints. She was lucky that these tests did not show some unrelated finding that would have required still more testing.

She is an example of how short-lived is the comforting effect of medical reassurance.

Moles and/or Malignant Melanoma

Newspapers explain at regular intervals that there is an increasing incidence of malignant melanoma, possibly as the result of the depletion of ozone in the atmosphere by man-made aerosols. Other kinds of skin cancer can be disfiguring, but only malignant melanoma is likely to be fatal. Furthermore, it is one of those few medical conditions that are completely curable in their early stages and not long after is almost always fatal. Therefore, it is sensible for everyone to take precautions against developing this disease and to take measures to insure that the condition is discovered early if it does indeed develop. Health worriers are likely to take these measures to an irrational extreme.

Amy had freckles and, perhaps, a somewhat greater number of moles than the average person. She had also had two or three bad sunburns when she was an adolescent. She read subsequently that even one bad sunburn predisposed to the likelihood of developing a melanoma. This possibility was increased further in people with a great number of moles. So, she decided to stay out of the sun. Such advice is commonly given; but Amy made a point of avoiding the sun in every season and even to the small extent she would be exposed to it during a walk. She felt nervous playing tennis or watching a baseball game. She never went out of doors on vacation without using sun block and insisting that everyone else in the family use it also. She interpreted advice to examine every part of her body for the appearance of a melanoma to mean that she should examine herself every week. She found herself looking at suspicious spots on her skin multiple times during the day even though she recognized that the spots could not have changed over the span of hours or minutes. Told by a dermatologist to come in once a year for a total body examination she found occasions to come in every few months. Often she asked about a particular mole which troubled her even though the dermatologist, and her regular physician too, had previously told her explicitly that that particular mole - sometimes only a mark - could never become malignant.

Amy had read about melanoma and recognized that a precautionary sign is a seemingly ordinary mole changing size or developing a variegation of pigment. Unfortunately, it <u>always</u> seemed to her that the mole she was currently concerned with was slightly larger than before or slightly darker. After one particular mole was deemed "suspicious" by her dermatologist, and removed, her preoccupation with her skin became crippling, despite the fact that the biopsy of the mole was read as negative.

<u>Good Things to Know</u>:

Sunburns are damaging to the skin and should be avoided if for no other reason than that they are painful. A lot of sunbathing year in and year out ages the skin prematurely. Sunbathing serves no useful purpose except in those particular times and places where a sun tan is thought attractive. But the danger of malignant melanoma is not made significantly worse by ordinary sun exposure. The compromise of the pleasures of life entailed by complete avoidance of sunlight is not justified by the minimal risk. In this context, Amy made the mistake often made by health worriers and by certain people who suffer form obsessive-compulsive disorder: they judge certain things known to be dangerous in considerable amounts or in certain circumstances to be dangerous always and even in insignificant amounts. They worry too much about germs, contamination and environmental poisons, many of which are present everywhere to some small extent. They do not understand the nature of risk. Sunlight, per se, is not dangerous. In fact, in those northern countries where the sun does not shine much, there is an increased rate of depression, alcoholism and certain vitamin deficiencies.

It is true, of course, that certain moles <u>do</u> appear suspicious. Sometimes even a trained dermatologist cannot tell by looking at a mole whether or not it has begun malignant transformation. These

222

moles are properly removed. <u>But the great majority of moles, freckles, and other skin flaws that health worriers agonize over bear no resemblance to anything potentially dangerous.</u> If the health worrier could look at those lesions and recognize immediately that they are harmless, he or she would break out of the habit of checking that keeps the worry wheel turning.

There is a cure for worrying excessively about malignant melanoma. It is to look at picture of various melanomas. The more pictures the better. Most of these pictures depict growths that could not be confused by any leap of the imagination with the particular marks or moles at the center of the health worrier's attention. As usual, it is difficult to get a health worrier to look at these scary pictures. Amy could be persuaded to do so only after a number of therapy sessions. But with long usage, these pictures become internalized and the next mole to be discovered suddenly can be dismissed out of mind just as quickly.

Similarly, women would be less likely to confuse menopause and ovarian cancer if they appreciated the wide range of irregular menses that occur routinely during menopause.

Men and women would worry less about mouth sores and oral cancer if they understood that cancers of the mouth tend to be hard and painless and, of course, persistent.

No one would be likely to worry about multiple sclerosis in the presence of sudden, shooting pains if it were understood that neuralgic pains of this sort are common and not a feature of multiple sclerosis.

Those people who worry about having contracted AIDS from a heterosexual partner many years ago would worry less if they understood how unlikely that possibility is. This devastating illness is caused by a fragile virus, easily destroyed outside of the body. The chance of an infected man communicating the disease to his wife after a full year of unprotected sexual intercourse is only 50%. The chance of an infected woman passing the disease to a male partner is even less. The chance of a nurse contracting the disease from the prick of a syringe full of HIV contaminated blood is less than 1 in 200.

Someone with an occasional bloody nose or bruises would be less likely to worry about leukemia if he or she understood that the bleeding that leukemia causes is persistent and widespread. People with enlarged lymph nodes would worry less about cancer if they understood, first of all, how frequently lymph nodes appear in association with viral infections and superficial skin infections and, secondly, that malignant lymph nodes tend to be large, sometimes matted, hard and adherent to surrounding tissues.

*   *   *

Doctors rely on such general descriptive rules to help diagnose medical illnesses; but these rules have many exceptions. They are only generally true. Just as each person is unique, the way a particular illness appears in a particular person is also unique. In order to make a final, accurate diagnosis, conflicting signs and symptoms must be weighed against each other. But time is on the doctor's side. Although an initial evaluation may point in the wrong direction, sooner or later the disease will manifest itself more characteristically and the correct diagnosis will become apparent.

Health worriers can usually find something to worry about. Physicians who have this emotional problem worry about diseases that no one else has ever heard of; but they do not worry about conditions which they know from their medical background do not fit with their symptoms. They do not worry about unicorns. Are they any better off? Certainly. Most physical symptoms are not worrisome to them. They can notice some lumps on their bodies without getting upset. This chapter then is an argument for knowing more.

It is not possible for a lay person to become as knowledgeable as a doctor no matter how much he or she reads. It is not sensible for patients to enter into quarrels with their physician on the basis of what they have read somewhere. But it is a plain fact that health wor-

224

riers have trouble believing everything that doctors tell them. Doctors tell them there is nothing to worry about, but they search the doctor's remarks (unwittingly — unwillingly) for the hidden problem, for the hint of something more serious, for the catch. It is this precise situation that can be relieved by knowing more. If health worriers cannot be comforted by reassuring remarks from their physician, they can at least confirm for themselves what the doctor has said. If, in fact, there is nothing to worry about, knowing more and more about the problem will make that more obvious, even to someone inclined by point of view to believe the worst.

Chapter Twelve: Dealing with Stress

It is often said that modern life is very stressful; and it is, although probably not any more stressful now than in the past — unless programming a VCR is more stressful than running into a bear at the back of the cave. Actually, the real stresses of life, I think, are more or less constant across the ages. Those concerns that preoccupy most people most of the time are the same that they have always been: making a living, maintaining a stable and satisfying relationship with a spouse, bringing up children successfully, and finding an advantageous place among the members of a particular community. Stress comes from difficulty pursuing these goals. Matters of health, also, have always worried people, although usually only at those times when good health seems to be at risk. When particular difficulties arise in any one of these areas, other concerns tend to fade. When health, or life itself, is threatened, all other problems tend to fade into insignificance. Consequently, health anxiety – a persistent worry about ill health - is very stressful to those who suffer from it.

Psychological stress, usually defined vaguely, is said to have all sorts of pernicious effects on physical health. Certainly, acute stress causes a variety of obvious bodily changes. They have been mentioned previously. Acid secretion rises in the stomach. Intestinal motility may speed up abruptly, or slow. Breathing and heart rate speed up. Blood pressure rises. Pupils dilate. The mouth becomes dry. Muscles tense. And so on. All of this is normal. There is a physiological purpose to all of these changes. They <u>enhance</u> the body's response to threat. Certain immunological changes also occur which may serve to improve the body's ability to ward off infection. Taken together these systemic changes do not cause illnesses, although they may worsen some that are already present. There is a continuing suspicion that a sudden shock, for example, may provoke a heart attack, but the evidence in support of this notion is not strong, and the effect, if it does exist, is not large. A small excess of cardiac deaths was reported during an earthquake in Japan; but that finding could have been the result only of heightened awareness during that period of time.

Although being anxious will not make anyone sick, it will cause changes of physiological function which may very well be construed by the health worrier as physical symptoms. It is important that these changes be understood for what they are, simply a consequence of arousal: the appropriate bodily response to danger. They are not a sign of illness. They may well be inappropriate to a particular situation, but only because some people, health worriers among them, perceive a danger in that situation when there is none.

Chronic stress is another story. I would like to be able to report to the reader an exact and accurate account of the risk to health that chronic stress presents; but the facts are hard to determine. The problem is not that the subject has not been studied. There have been literally thousands of medical reports addressing this question. Most of them have found chronic stress to have a significant, unfavorable influence on health. The difficulty lies in determining how credible these studies are.

Medical research reports in general cannot be taken at face value. The results of any scientific investigation are only more or less valid depending on many factors, including the design of the experiment, the statistical analyses, the volume and reliability of the data, and the prejudices of the investigators. Often, conflicting studies are published simultaneously. Sometimes it is plain to a knowledgeable reader that a particular study is defective. The number of subjects may be too small to support the statistical conclusion. The population tested may not be appropriate. The study may not be "blinded" properly, allowing placebo effects and the prior presumptions of the investigator to contaminate the experimental findings. Sometimes other confounding factors are present. Good studies should control for extraneous influences such as diet or the concomitant use of drugs of one sort or another. Many times, however, a particular study seems to have been done carefully. It may have been published in a prestigious journal which is known to require careful peer review before an article is accepted for publication. The results described may lend robust support to the hypothesis being tested. It is a convincing study. And yet subsequent studies testing the same idea show progressively less definite results, and then, finally, some definitive study comes along explicitly contradicting the original. This pattern repeats itself more often than is ordinarily supposed and is the reason why doctors are not inclined to jump on any bandwagon. They are conservative. They hesitate, for example, to substitute a novel treatment for one that is more conventional unless a number of studies confirming each other make that change imperative. By that time, they usually seem to be dragging their feet. Sometimes they do, in fact, wait longer than they should to accept new ways of considering medical problems, especially if doing so entails a so-called paradigm shift.

In the context of medicine, a paradigm shift means a radical new way of considering a disease, rather than the usual bit by bit advance in understanding or in treatment. For example, peptic u1cers were discovered a few years ago to be <u>infectious</u> in origin in the majority of cases. This idea was so revolutionary, it has not been fully integrated yet in the management of that illness. In this case, the basic conservatism of the medical community has slowed progress. Their inveterate skepticism has prevented them also from recognizing the documented advantages of vitamins in preventing a half-dozen serious medical problems. They come to that skepticism, however, for good reason. There is a long history of half-baked claims for vitamin therapy. These claims have misled practitioners and patients over the years with serious consequences. For one thing, it is possible to overdose on certain vitamins. Certain minerals added routinely to vitamins may hurt rather than help. Besides, there is the basic issue of knowing the truth of a particular scientific conjecture before recommending a treatment on that basis. When is a particular idea documented sufficiently to recommend to patients a new drug – or, especially, a new way of living? How much evidence should one have before recommending that people change their diet? For the reasons given, it is difficult to know exactly how much confidence one should invest in a particular piece of medical research.

The research on the effects of stress is especially unclear. For purposes of these studies acute stress is usually defined arbitrarily in terms of a contrived situation — such as asking someone to sort objects under pressure, or the like — much removed from the real stresses of life, such as marital conflict or being fired from a job. Even then, the extent of the stress differs widely from one individual to another depending on other circumstances in that person's life. Losing a job, for instance, has a different impact depending on the professional credentials of the affected person, his or her age, previous experience of being fired, other work options, and, especially, self-confidence, which is the distillate of every other prior experience.

Some people seem to be under tremendous pressure from experiences other people would regard as trivial. A leaky sink can and does cause turmoil in someone who is exquisitely vulnerable for some special reason — in one case that I know of because of a fear of interlopers, such as plumbers. Waiting on line is very stressful for most phobics. Some people take criticism philosophically and with good grace; others become very upset.

It is surprising that conditions such as panic disorder or depression are marked by very few long-term physical effects. People with panic attacks have a very slightly elevated risk for coronary artery disease after a period of 20 or 30 years. Possibly. Some individuals who have been judged to be depressive in temperament have a slightly elevated risk of cancer once again over a period of decades. Even the well-known association between the Type A personality - angry and impatient - and heart disease is not entirely certain. There is one study, for instance, among the thousands on this subject that suggests that having had one heart attack, someone with Type A personality is <u>less</u> likely to have another. And Type A persons do not usually report that they are feeling stress. Contrary to conventional wisdom there is very little real evidence that <u>acute</u> stress has any discernible, <u>significant</u> effect on health. Every once in a while a study appears that suggests that people who are under stress are somewhat more likely to catch cold. Possibly. But this much is certain: the increase in heart rate and breathing associated with being nervous does not make people sick, even if it persists for hours and days. The increase in stomach acid secretion associated with stress does not cause ulcers in those who are not predisposed to ulcers for other reasons. The physiological effects of being nervous disappear without trace when the period of being nervous is followed, as it is, inevitably, by a period of being not nervous.

Most studies about the physical effects of chronic stress are simple correlations. When an association is found between chronic anxiety and subsequent heart disease, for example, it is not clear whether the anxiety is <u>causing</u> the heart disease, or whether <u>some underlying vulnerability is causing both</u>. It is not usually clear whether alleviating one will lessen the danger of the other. Intervention studies, which are designed to discover precisely that, are subject to distortion by placebo effects. In other words, the simple act of offering a therapy, any therapy, causes people to get better, especially if the doctors or therapists administering the treatment believe in its effectiveness.

When beneficial effects on health are reported by studies purporting to reduce stress, the results are hard to interpret since the same studies have usually encouraged subjects also to lose weight, change their diet, and exercise too, all at the same time. When the illness concerned is coronary artery disease, the principal benefits are likely to come from a diet that lowers saturated fat and cholesterol and from exercise, rather than from stress reduction. All these confounding factors make it difficult to tease out the effects of stress per se on the body. It is good to keep in mind these hidden complications when reading a facile account in a newspaper of the latest medical studies on stress, or on any other subject. For one thing, negative results are rarely reported and yet are just as important in understanding any scientific question.

The conventional wisdom is that emotional stress over a period of years increases the danger of a variety of illnesses, including stroke, heart disease, and cancer. Having stated my reservations about accepting some of the evidence reported in this connection, I should say also that I think, probably, that the conventional wisdom is correct. There is very likely an influence of emotional stress over time on physical health — but that influence is probably <u>not</u> as great as it is often made out to be. Certainly it is not as devastating as cigarette smoking. Health worriers, who by definition worry too much about their health, tend to worry also about the effect their worrying itself has on their health. They worry, and they worry about worrying, which is why they are likely to read a book such as this. The effects of stress are real enough to justify an attempt to diminish them. Such an effort would be justified in any case simply because stress is unpleasant- and often avoidable.

For our purposes, stress may be regarded as a set of circumstances that cause a particular person to become upset. As suggested earlier, the circumstances themselves are rarely so dramatic that it can be assumed automatically that the person <u>must</u> be experiencing stress. Whether or not there is stress and how severe it is depends on the individual. <u>Some</u> people are <u>not</u> threatened by:

1. Quarreling with a boss.
2. Missing a deadline.
3. Attempting an assignment beyond their capacity.
4. Going on a job interview.
5. Speaking publicly to a large group of people.
6. Backing the car into the garage doors.
7. Confronting a full-field audit by the IRS.

8. Losing an envelope which contained one thousand dollars of somebody else's money.
9. Studying for a qualifying examination.
10. Cooking for a party of twelve
11. Coping with three sick children at the same time.
12. Being passed over for a promotion.
13. Serving in the army.
14. Listening to customers complain constantly.
15. Having in-laws visit for a week or two.
16. Rushing for a fraternity.
17. Being pregnant.
18. Being married to someone who is pregnant.
19. Making too little money.
20. Moving to a new city.

Even

21. Being sick.

I have seen <u>some</u> people manage these situations gracefully and comfortably, sometimes joyfully. I have seen <u>no one</u> who is immune to all of these circumstances, or, indeed, most of them. Similarly, I have seen others falter and complain bitterly of the stress of:

1. Having to get up each morning to go to work.
2. Dieting.
3. Checking their children's homework.
4. Quarreling with a friend.
5. Cleaning the bathroom.
6. Going on vacation.
7. Dating.

Perhaps there are certain experiences so inherently distressing it may be presumed that <u>everyone</u> in that situation is feeling stress, even when that person seems on the surface to be calm:

1. Losing a spouse through death or divorce.
2. Killing someone, even when the person doing so is a policeman.

3. Going to jail.
4. Serving in the military in combat.
5. Being hospitalized, or raped, or assaulted.
6. Getting fired.
7. Being seriously injured in an automobile accident.

And, certainly,

8. Being very sick or having a child who is very sick.

These traumatic situations do not lend themselves readily to scientific investigation. There is some convincing evidence that severe trauma can lead to serious and long-lasting psychological changes, the so-called post-traumatic stress disorder. This condition demands treatment. Thankfully these situations occur infrequently and, when they do, most people manage to live through them, and after a period of time return to the person they used to be.

Most people, however, are under stress because of particular attitudes they have towards themselves. These ideas color their experiences. They are stressed, and sometimes just plain frightened, not because of the situation they find themselves in, but because of the way they construe that situation. Certain emotional problems characteristically cause stress in situations experienced by most other people as benign.

If someone considers himself incompetent, he will feel pressure whenever he is required to perform some difficult task. More than other people, he will anticipate failing. He is likely to interpret that failure, if it does come, as a public confirmation of just how inept he is. He is embarrassed and demoralized by a circumstance that most other people would regard as inevitable from time to time and inconsequential. Such a person would find stressful any of the following situations:

1. Beginning a new job.
2. Being promoted.
3. Working under a deadline.

4. Being criticized by a boss.
5. Making complicated arrangements for a vacation or for a wedding.
6. Working without guidelines.

    – and dozens of other situations, particularly at work, which other people might find difficult at worst, but also interesting and maybe even exciting. These other people do not regard falling short, if that should happen, as a statement about their overall abilities.

    If someone considers herself to be unattractive or unappealing, a different set of experiences become stressful, but for similar reasons:

1. A blind date.
2. Going to a party where she knows only a few people.
3. Any activity for singles.
4. Spending a few days alone.
5. Going to the beach or to an exercise class.
6. Shopping for clothes.

    If someone is afraid of conflict, she may have an inordinate need to please. These situations, then, will be stressful:

1. Working for two bosses.
2. Trying to satisfy simultaneously the demands of work and family.
3. Dealing with demanding people in general.
4. Refusing favors when asked by friends.
5. Getting into an argument with a salesperson.

    If someone feels inferior, having to express an opinion — any sort of opinion – becomes stressful. Meeting with a child's teacher is threatening. Making a mistake, even the possibility of making a mistake – <u>any</u> kind of mistake – becomes threatening. The need to be liked makes any social interaction potentially threatening. The need to present a good appearance to everyone may make the simple act of getting dressed in the morning threatening. <u>Stress, then, is as much a statement of a particular vulnerability as it is a particular circumstance.</u> The less self-confidence a person has, the more situations are likely to be experienced as stressful.

How then does one cope with stress?

An attractive and capable woman had achieved a senior position in a bank at a time when banking presented special hurdles for women. She was, in general, self-confident; but her confidence did not extend to her relationships with men. These took on a stereotyped form. Typically, she would meet a man and quickly grow attached to him and just as quickly begin to wonder what the man thought about her. What did he really mean when he said, "I'll see you?" Is he seeing someone else too? Should I check to see if his car is parked in front of his office? Should I come right out and ask him what his intentions are? Am I coming across as too clinging? More often than not, the relationship would fall apart in a matter of weeks; and within a month or so she was in a similar relationship with another man and asking the same questions. The stress of undertaking these troubled relationships, one after the other, took its toll. Besides suffering the distracting preoccupations described above, she had trouble eating and sleeping and often found herself pacing restlessly.

In order to address her emotional problems, she entered into a kind of relaxation therapy marked by deep breathing exercises and assuming the lotus position!

Is this a sensible response to her problem? Even if breathing deeply makes her feel good all over, will this help her to deal more effectively with men? Is it not more reasonable to address the root causes of her stress?

I knew someone once who used to drive around curves at high speed and as a result had wrecked three cars in potentially life-threatening accidents. Recognizing grudgingly the danger in the manner of his driving, he resolved to buy tires with better traction!

Is this an adequate response? I think not. Really good tires with really good treads might help a little to prevent a future accident, but not to the extent of driving sensibly.

The woman described above found the ordinary and often pleasurable business of dating very stressful. Maybe the unpleasant effects of stress could be relieved to some extent by yoga; but surely she would do better by removing the causes of her stress. What were they?

A hierarchy of Bad Ideas led her to anticipate a threat to her self-esteem when no such threat was likely. First of all, obviously, she expected to be rejected by men. Less obvious, at least to her, were the reasons underlying that belief. These were other beliefs:

1. That she was unattractive.
2. That she was too "available" to men.
3. That she could not be interesting to a man for any length of time.
4. That men were unreliable.
5. That men were threatened by successful women like her.
6. That men were less inclined than women to settle into a monogamous relationship.

And so on.

These are not easy ideas to change, but that is the purpose of psychotherapy, and that is the reason why psychotherapy takes so long. It is much easier to assume the lotus position (perhaps this is too glib; I, for one, find it impossible to get into the lotus position.)

Similar Bad Ideas lie behind most stressful situations. Changing those ideas about the world and about oneself is critical to lessening that stress permanently. Imagine, for one example, an employee who is confident of his skills and his ability to find a new job if necessary, who is not afraid of authority figures in general and his boss in particular, whose job is not fundamental to his self-esteem, at least no more than his place in his family and in his community, and who feels that he is, in most people's opinion, worthwhile. Such a person is not likely to find any job stressful.

Granted that changes in attitude are the most effective way of coping with stress, is there at least some benefit in the usual remedy of relaxation exercises? Probably. In the same sense that buying good tires lessen the risk of driving too fast. There is little, though, to recommend one system of relaxation techniques over another.

Relaxation exercises:

1. Sit in a comfortable chair. Close your eyes. Concentrate on relaxing the muscles of your face, then your neck muscles, then the muscles of your upper limbs and then your lower limbs. Then do it all over again.

2. Concentrate on your breathing and on the beating of your heart. Try to discover a hidden rhythm. Some practitioners recommend detailed breathing exercises to cope with panic attacks. These work, not because breathing properly counteracts anxiety, but because their technique for breathing properly requires such attention to detail that someone attempting it is distracted inevitably from the panic attack, which only lasts for a few moments anyway. In this regard, it works about as well as trying to say, "Peter Piper picked a peck of pickled peppers 10 times" in a row without making a mistake.

3. Sit in a comfortable chair. Close your eyes. Try to relax. Ponder nothingness. Empty your mind as far as you can of all thoughts and certainly those thoughts that preoccupy you most of the time. Hum to yourself, or think of a nonsense word with no connotations: a number, or your name, or a nonsense syllable. Contrary to what some people say, the nonsense word does not have to be chosen carefully with our own particular personality in mind. This process is called "meditation," even though meditation originally implied thinking about something, not thinking about nothing. Experienced meditators claim that the beneficial effects improve with practice. Some claim that they can levitate. Self-hypnosis falls somewhere in this category.

4. Exercise, oddly enough, if it takes on a repetitive, mindless character, such as pedaling a stationery bicycle, is said to achieve the same beneficial mental state as relaxation exercises.

5. Try Yoga, which is a systematic set of exercises for attaining control over body and mind. A variety of health benefits have been attributed to yoga, which has been around for centuries and, perhaps for that reason, deserves at least some credence.

6. Sleep. Taking a nap has been shown to provide many of the benefits attributed to relaxation in general. In fact, studies have shown that some meditators at the very moment they think they are levitating are actually asleep. This is my preferred method of relaxation.

In order for any of these exercises to be helpful, they should be entered into in a spirit of optimism which, it is plain to the reader, I find hard to justify. Their effects, if any, are transitory. Relaxation exercises are not an integral part of the program reported in this book. Still, many people report that they are helped by them. If you want to train yourself to relax in this manner, you should leave some time every day, a half-hour perhaps, or longer, to participate in such a program. As a symbolic statement of the wish to re-think the course of one's life, it may serve a special purpose. Stepping away from the frantic demands of work or the headlong pace of family routine for even a short time every day is a way of saying that certain activities have less urgency and less importance than we ordinarily attribute to them. Even taking out time to read a book quietly may serve such a purpose.

Thought Stopping

Relaxation exercises may be regarded as an attempt to control feeling states directly, without special regard to the person's circumstances. Since emotional states in general <u>are</u> a response to circumstances – at least <u>perceived</u> circumstances – this is hard to accomplish. Drugs are another attempt to manage feelings directly; and they have usefulness in varying degrees, for the treatment of mood disorders in particular. (See the sections on drugs in this book.) Since feelings are interwoven inextricably with certain thoughts, such as the Bad Ideas referred to throughout this book, cognitive therapists have tried to alter feelings by altering thoughts, sometimes in ways that do not require reasoning with the patient. Yelling "stop" into their ears is such a way. It has been attempted as a way of interrupting the persistent ruminations that characterize health anxiety and other obsessional disorders. But thoughts too, no less than feelings, are an automatic response to the experiences someone has had. The same thoughts return stubbornly. Reasoning with patients, if that means simply lecturing to them, is also not effective. Telling a person to look on the bright side will not cause him to become less depressed. However, that person should, and in many cases, can learn to look more accurately at himself and at the world and find reason to become more cheerful. Someone troubled by health anxiety needs to have in place strategies for finding out the truth about his or her condition in order to worry less. Still, once again, it would be nice if these repetitive thoughts could somehow be blotted out directly. Indeed, <u>briefly</u>, they can.

One evening, when I was in my college dormitory room, I had a panic attack. It was not my first, but they were still new to me. I was overcome by the sudden sense of urgency which is the defining sensation of this unpleasant experience. I thought I was going crazy. I couldn't think about anything other than my rising sense of panic. Since my heart — in fact, my whole body — was racing, I thought what I should do is jump up and down or run around. So I did jump off the couch I had been lying on. I ran down three flights of stairs, ran around the block, ran up the three flights of stairs and threw myself back down on the couch so hard I pounded my head up against the wall. A few minutes later, when the pain had subsided enough to think clearly, I realized the panic attack and the thoughts I had been thinking had vanished. So, I had discovered something interesting: given enough pain I could distract myself from whatever I had been thinking, no matter how compelling the thought!

It turns out that if someone is similarly obsessed by thoughts of contamination, let's say, or by the thought of cancer, that person can be distracted temporarily by somebody else yelling "stop" at him. To some extent, patients in a program of "thought-stopping" can train themselves to yell "stop" inwardly at themselves.

It is possible with practice to learn to distract oneself from a particular thought, but certain thoughts are more pressing than others: It is easier to run away from consideration of what to have for dinner, than to put aside the thought of being fatally ill. Even with practice thoughts can be managed actively for only brief periods of time. Unwanted thoughts creep back in willy-nilly. In the treatment of panic disorder, brief periods of time are enough. A panic attack results from an abnormal focus on one's mind and body that lasts at its most extreme only for moments. Any measure than can focus attention elsewhere - short of pounding one's head against the wall - will lessen that distress and with practice can dispel the attack altogether.

Health anxiety is another matter. The concerns that trouble the health worrier are varied and persist in one form or another for years. Simply turning one's mind away for a time does not help. Psychological contrivances of this sort or of any sort suggest a kind of magic by which people can be made well without real effort. In the end, unnecessary worry about health or about anything else can be dispelled only by a better understanding of the substance of those concerns: by learning the facts, by determining what is real. If there is a real danger, cautionary steps can be taken; if there is no real danger, that fact becomes apparent, finally, even to someone who starts out inclined to worry. In such a way, the unnecessary stress of health worry can be subtracted from all the other stresses of life. The trick is how to deal with particular stresses, not stress in general.

Drugs

Another means, besides relaxation exercises, by which physicians attempt to relieve anxiety directly, without bothering to discover or counter the underlying reasons for the anxiety, is through the

240

use of tranquilizers. The very word "tranquil" calls up to my mind a picture of someone sitting calmly in a cushiony, high-back chair before a crackling fire, wearing a soft, silken dressing gown and sipping a brandy, possibly listening to music. Feeling tranquil from time to time is desirable, although only from time to time in a world where excitement and adventure are also possible. It is depressing to discover that there are many people whose appreciation of life is so meager that their principal aspiration is to become tranquil. In fairness, though, there are many others who would like to enjoy life actively but who are worried or anxious so continuously that they seem never to be tranquil. That they should seek some respite by any means at all is understandable.

For the sake of discussion, let us imagine that tomorrow morning a new drug for anxiety comes on the market. So far, this is not hard to imagine since new anxiolytics are introduced frequently. The market is lucrative and none of the very many drugs currently prescribed work really well. This new drug, however, is different. It is the perfect tranquilizer. Unlike all the others, it has no side effects. It is non-sedating and, therefore, not likely to interfere with learning or driving an automobile. It does not cause excessive sleepiness. Old people are not endangered by this drug. People taking it do not get high, and, consequently, it does not encourage abuse. Tolerance does not develop and neither does addiction. There is no interaction with other drugs. Although the drug is appearing for the first time tomorrow, we have been assured by a well-known psychic that it will be safe even after 20 or 30 years of continuous use. Furthermore, the drug works unfailingly. Whatever the circumstances, in the face of fire and flood, not to mention ill-health, this drug induces a state of calm. Also it is cheap. Would we want to use this drug every day? Do we want always to be calm? Is there no good reason, ever, to be anxious? Of course, there is.

The sense of anxiety is part of a complicated psychological and physiological response to danger. Human beings have evolved this adaptation. In other words, the subjective feeling of anxiety may be unpleasant, but it is necessary for survival. We are <u>supposed</u> to be anxious the night before an examination or a job interview, or in the face of fire or flood. Someone who is calm and comfortable in such circumstances is not likely to think quickly or to move quickly or adroitly, or to plan effectively, or to act with that extra effort that often makes the difference between success and failure. Someone studying for an examination will work more tirelessly, more alertly and with greater focus by virtue of his or her being anxious. Those who are anxious about their health are similarly at an advantage if they are, in fact, sick or in danger of becoming sick. They are then more likely than they would be otherwise to exercise properly, eat properly and in other ways take care of themselves, including seeking medical care promptly. A sensible physician would not want to prescribe this remarkable new tranquilizer to ordinary people reacting to the ordinary stresses of life.

But is it possible to be <u>too</u> anxious? Yes, but really only under two kinds of circumstances. The first situation occurs frequently: a problem which in most people's eyes is not very threatening is, nevertheless, worrisome to a particular person because he or she has misunderstood the situation. Sometimes the cause is simple ignorance. A man is afraid of a bridge falling down in a high wind when no such thing can happen. A woman is afraid of catching AIDS from shaking hands with a homosexual when, in fact, the disease cannot be transmitted in such a way. Sometimes someone has a particular reason to be afraid. Some of these reasons have been described previously as a cause of stress. They lie hidden in the character of the individual. Here, one misapprehension may be piled on another. Someone fearing unrealistically that he or she may have offended someone else becomes unduly anxious and may be made more anxious by the equally unrealistic thought that the offended party will retaliate in some way – and, perhaps, that everyone else who matters will also be offended at some similar unintended slight and withdraw

242

also, leaving that man or woman alone forever. Someone so afraid throughout so many different encounters will seem anxious most of the time to everyone — too anxious, since the reasons are not apparent. Sooner or later, as likely as not, such an anxious person may be given tranquilizers. Many such people take these drugs for years with only temporary relief, and often not much of that. A better remedy, I think, although more difficult, is to make plain those distortions of perception and thought that cause people in the first place to become so persistently and unnecessarily afraid.

The second circumstance in which someone may reasonably be said to be "too anxious" occurs when that person is suffering an illness which causes anxiety directly. There are a number of such illnesses, some of which have traditionally been considered mental or emotional in origin, such as depression, and others which are ordinarily considered organic, but which have psychological manifestations. These include neurological and endocrine disorders and drug reactions. And there are many others. Anyone can develop any one of these conditions. Someone so affected may become anxious however clear-eyed and resilient he or she might be ordinarily. The subjective sense of being anxious is driven internally in these cases rather than by any threatening circumstances. Such a person may need medicine to get better depending on the underlying condition. Tranquilizers may not be the best treatment.

This, then is the difference: someone who is anxious because of a perceived danger, real or imaginary, needs to learn how to cope with that danger. In the case of health anxiety, there is, by definition, no real danger; and the health worrier needs primarily to learn how to develop a perspective which allows that fact to become clear. Drugs, in my opinion, have very little effect on this problem <u>unless the health worrier is suffering also from an overlapping illness for which medication is the appropriate treatment.</u> In those cases where medication is appropriate, such as depression, it is usually critical.

There are therapists who feel more comfortable with psychological interventions and will try drugs only when such treatment is shown not to work; there are other physicians who find it easier to give drugs, usually with a nod to "cost-effectiveness" or out of a real conviction that psychological interventions are unscientific and unlikely to work. They refer their patients for cognitive-behavioral therapies only when the drugs do not work. Neither approach can be justified by what is known about the anxiety disorders. Depending on particular circumstances there is a place both for psychological therapies and for the use of drugs, and often for both together. Which treatment is primary depends on the distinctions drawn above.

Having drawn that distinction between anxiety which can be spoken of loosely as psychological in origin and that which has a physiological cause, I would like to blur that distinction. In real life it is not always easy to tell one from the other. And one sometimes leads to the other. And they can overlap. And, in principle, at least, a psychological illness might just as well be treated by a drug as by a psychological intervention. Those conditions for which that might be true are discussed in <u>Worried Sick? The Workbook</u>. Still, in the end, health anxiety, being essentially an idea, can be displaced only by a better idea. This book is intended to dispel those Bad Ideas about health that cause the health worrier to worry unnecessarily. It is a strategy for finding out the truth.

A few words about the psychosomatic diseases:

For reasons that are more or less arbitrary the American Psychiatric Association classifies hypochondriasis together with the psychosomatic disorders. Both conditions have to do with symptoms referable to the human body. By that standard they might just as well have included hearing loss and tooth decay. Hypochondriasis should have been included among the anxiety disorders. Psychosomatic diseases include asthma, peptic ulcers, ulcerative colitis, essential hypertension, certain skin conditions, and, depending on who is writing about them, rheumatoid arthritis and various other conditions. The medical literature concerning them is considerable and mostly wrong. One school of thought used to explain them as manifestations of particular personality types. People developed stomach ulcers if they were passive and dependent. Another school explained them as manifestations of particular emotional conflicts, mostly unconscious. Someone might develop a rash if people "got under his skin." Colitis, which is marked by diarrhea, was a "weeping colon", a displacement to the colon by people who could not cry. Someone who was in conflict about expressing anger would develop arthritis so she "couldn't make a fist." There was a time when these explanations, which had a kind of nitwit charm, had a considerable grip on the psychiatric mind. Consequently, patients were blamed for their illnesses. They were taught to feel guilty about feeling sick; and they were psychoanalyzed sometimes for years with no noticeable effect on the course of their physical illnesses.

There are some points worth making about the psychosomatic disorders:

1. Anyone who is chronically ill - and these are all long-term disorders that wax and wane unpredictably - may very well develop personality problems. It is not surprising that someone who is always sick becomes disagreeable or withdrawn-or depressed. So much is true for health worriers too.

2. These are all disease with complicated organic causes. They are not caused psychologically, but psychological distress does worsen many of them, probably because of the effects of stress on the immune system. Health worriers should not worry about worrying themselves into one of these disorders.

Chapter Thirteen: The Role of the Family

Cynthia had always thought of herself as a worrier. She came from a family of worriers. Her father worried about the weather. Her mother's worries were more diffuse. She worried about money and about additives in food and about the possibility of Cynthia contracting a venereal disease although she knew her daughter was still a virgin at the age of 24. And she too worried about the weather. Bad weather threatened in ways that were hard to define, including not only the dangers of driving in the rain and snow, but also the vague possibility of being trapped somewhere alone and far away from home, such as at a friend's house on the other side of town. Cold weather was considered dangerous to health; and Cynthia's mother was wont to hide a scarf surreptitiously in Cynthia's briefcase in case a cold front came though while she was at work. Cynthia worried most of all about the difficulty in this day and age of meeting a suitable, gentlemanly-sort of man with whom she could settle down and raise a family; but not far behind were health worries.

Cynthia's health worries had become aggravated recently when she developed hives. The hives appeared in crops every day for a period of months. No cause for them had been discovered.

"A lot of bad diseases can cause hives," Cynthia's mother told her, not entirely in error. A great many illnesses of all sorts cause hives, although most cases of this common and usually benign condition appear and then disappear without their cause ever becoming apparent. "Aunt Charlotte got hives before she died," she added some time later. "It was the first sign, I think. We didn't know it then. Of course, that has nothing to do with your hives."

Cynthia was upset even before listening to her mother's remarks. She watched apprehensively while her hives faded each day only to reappear the next day or the day after. Sometimes there seemed a reason; something she ate perhaps. Other times they would simply return for no discernible reason. And they itched. The doctors whom she consulted told her she probably had some kind of allergy and "not to worry." She worried nevertheless. One doctor patted her on the shoulder and told her she would be all right "unless" she developed hives on her larynx, which might kill her but which was "very, very unlikely."

Various medications were prescribed for Cynthia, including anti-histamines, which lessened the itching, but did not prevent further outbreaks of hives. When she seemed to her physician to become increasingly anxious and depressed, he prescribed an anti-depressant also - to which her mother objected, however, on grounds that it would affect her mind. In fact, her mother had a number of strong opinions about Cynthia's medical care. At various times she told her:

"I don't want you taking this drug" (the anti-depressant) "it causes homicidal tendencies." (It does not.)

"I don't think you should listen to this guy, he's not a rash specialist." (He was, in fact, a dermatologist.)

"They should be able to figure out what's causing these things." (Again, usually not so in the case of hives.)

"You should stay home from work and rest more. Take a nap." (Naps do not have a salutary effect on hives.)

"Your hives are going to get worse in the cold." (Sometimes true!)

"Stay away from salty food." (Good advice for those who are inclined to hypertension, but not relevant to the treatment of hives.)

A drama played out every day in which Cynthia and her mother upset each other, each expressing some concern that had not occurred to the other. Also, they entered into the practice of examining Cynthia's skin, Cynthia relying on her mother to determine, in those areas which she herself could not inspect comfortably, whether her hives were just a little bit better or a little bit worse.

Cynthia often described her mother as sympathetic and "supportive;" but, in fact, their relationship contributed to her growing concern about her hives and about her health in general. And that inclination to worry long outlasted this particular, relatively minor, illness.

*   *   *

Tom, on the other hand, could not have described his family as sympathetic. "They don't understand," was the way he put it. Perhaps because his illness had no obvious physical manifestations, such as a skin rash, they dismissed his complaints out of hand.

Over the years Tom had developed a number of definite, diagnosable illnesses, including hypothyroidism and Lyme disease; but at the age of 47 his principal physical symptom was of severe pain on one side of the body. According to one of the number of neurologists he had seen, he had an "impossible" pain since it involved the left side of his entire face including his tongue and also his left arms and leg, a distribution of pain not explainable by any conceivable anatomical lesion. The neurologist seemed to take offense at having been asked his medical opinion of such a patient, as if Tom had been purposely dissembling. Other doctors were more charitable, and a number gave one or another explanation for Tom's condition, but none of the remedies prescribed were helpful.

When Tom, on occasion, took to bed because of back pain, his children would sigh audibly and roll their eyes, as if to say, "There he goes again." His wife was more explicit: "It's all in your head, for God's sake," she said. When he mused aloud about the possibility of his having a brain tumor, or worsening chronic Lyme disease, she told him that there was nothing the matter with him. "If you keep crying 'wolf,' " she pointed out, "no one is going to believe you when you're really sick." She had not always been so unsympathetic.

In the first years of their marriage, Tom's wife listened with concern to all of his worries, including those that centered on his health. When he seemed sick, she comforted him. When he got well quickly, or proved never to have been sick in the first place, she pointed out to him in a good-natured way that those dire consequences he had imagined never really came about. The fact that he had not developed cancer in the past, however, seemed to have no impact on whatever fears he had currently. He asked vague, stereotyped questions: "Do you think I have bags under my eyes?" "Do I look pale?" Her replies, however encouraging, were unconvincing to him. They did not stop him from asking the same question a few minutes later. Naturally, inevitably perhaps, her responses became perfunctory.

Tom: Do I look pale?

His wife, reading a book: You look fine.

Tom: You're not listening to me.

His wife, still reading: Yes, I am.

Asked the same questions day after day, and eventually year after year, Tom's wife replied with growing annoyance and sometimes ridicule. Their children, now old enough to enjoy a joke at their father's expense, joined in. Tom's marriage, which was marked also at other times for other reasons with increasing ill-will, ended in divorce. His worsening health anxiety was one factor.

*   *   *

Family members have considerable influence on any one among them who is troubled by health anxiety, or any other emotional problem, for that matter. They can make things better, or worse. In fact, as each family is unique, the psychodynamics of each operate in complicated ways to both good and bad effect. The families described above, although well-meaning, at least initially, illustrate the kinds of interaction that serve to aggravate health worries. It is easy for a family member to do and say just those very things that cause a health worrier to focus still greater attention on his or her health. This trap can be avoided. It is important, also, to resist the urge to turn away altogether on the theory that there is nothing to be done. Handling the exaggerated concerns of a health worrier properly makes a difference in outcome. Put simply, doing the wrong thing makes their anxieties worse, doing the right thing diminishes them.

The following are guidelines for friends and family to follow in coping with someone troubled by health anxiety. They parallel the recommendations for patients made in previous chapters.

Do not:

1. Ridicule the health worrier. Naturally. If health worriers become more distressed for any reason, they react physically as one does usually to stress: with pain, including stomachaches, headaches and backaches, with insomnia, palpitations, loss of appetite, and so on. They are likely then to focus still more fixedly on their physical symptoms. In that respect a human being is like a bell. Struck by any sort of blow, the bell gives off the same sound. A person who is compulsive, for example, becomes more so if depressed or made more anxious than usual by circumstances. A phobic person becomes more phobic. Someone who is paranoid becomes still more suspicious. No matter what upsets a health worrier, whether it is a problem at work, for example, or criticism by a family member, that person is likely to respond by worrying more about his or her health. Besides, being made to feel ridiculous is demoralizing in general. Such a person finds it harder to admit to any weakness and consequently is less likely to identify himself as a health worrier and will be less likely to seek help. It is a good idea, in any case, not to make fun of other people since we are all ridiculous in someone's eyes.

2. Do not collaborate in the health worrier's compulsive checking. Repetitious checking accomplishes nothing. It elicits no useful information and serves only to focus more attention on the health worrier's fears. Do not express an opinion on whether he or she looks a little better or worse. Do not make a judgment on whether or not a lump or a skin lesion has changed size overnight. Without medical training these judgments are unreliable. Besides, such subtle changes usually have no clinical significance. Do not offer routine reassurance. This is another form of

checking. Telling someone who is frightened not to worry does not work. Empty phrases, such as "You'll be fine," or "You look better today," are not helpful. Resist the health worrier's prodding to get such reassurance. Explain that your not answering is not a sign of indifference, but that you are <u>not supposed to answer</u>. Giving the same responses to the same questions over and over again is not convincing.

If telling health worriers that they look a little better does not comfort them, telling them that they look a little worse is certainly not a good idea! If you yourself are a health worrier,[1] you may be able to imagine catastrophes that have not yet occurred to them. Do not suggest these to them. Health worriers are much more inclined by point of view to believe in bad news than good. It is best not to comment one way or the other.

3. <u>Do not profess a medical opinion.</u> Do not diagnose. Do not propose medical treatments for illnesses you do not understand. Do not recommend particular drugs on the basis of personal experience. A medication that worked for you is not necessarily a good choice for your spouse or your child. You would not suggest to them that they wear your eyeglasses. Especially do not recommend herbal remedies. Some of them do indeed have pharmacological effects of one sort or another. Because of a quirk of law, no governmental authority analyzes these products. On occasion they have been found to be laced with tranquilizers and other drugs. Herbal concoctions purported to be of one particular type are produced by different manufacturers and have different potencies. Sometimes the potency varies from batch to batch even when produced by the same manufacturer. Herbal products are not harmless! They are also no more "natural" than many

---

[1] This is a condition, after all, that runs in families. It reflects views usually held in common, like being a Democrat or a Republican, or a Presbyterian.

drugs, some of which were derived initially from plants or animals. Besides, natural substances are not inherently safer than those made by man. Not counting the familiar poisons produced by mushrooms and many other plants, ordinary foods, including vegetables, which are on balance good for us, have carcinogens in amounts greatly exceeding those routinely added to foods in the form of preservatives. This is not a reason to avoid vegetables. It is an argument in favor of judging each substance on its own merits and avoiding those, natural or not, whose effectiveness and whose dangers, have not been determined.

There is also sold to the public a class of presumably medicinal agents which are known, as well as anything can be known, to be ineffective. Among them are homeopathic drugs which are based, literally, on a kind of magic and whose formulation is contrary to fundamental scientific principles.

Do not conclude on the basis of what you have read in newspapers that certain drugs are dangerous or better than or worse than other drugs. See Chapter 2 on drugs. Do not offer these ill-considered opinions to the health worrier, who is likely to react in an exaggerated manner to the drug, or to refuse it altogether at a time when taking it may be important, even critical. Similarly, do not venture negative opinions on certain treatment modalities such as electric shock therapy or other procedures such as Caesarean section as if they are never indicated no matter what the circumstances. Do not repeat absurd generalizations such as "surgeons always like to cut." Or "Psychiatrists want to keep you in therapy forever." They make health worriers more afraid of seeking medical help and more distrusting of doctors than they are already.

Do not find fault with the health worrier's current physician unless you have good reason. If someone develops an illness that is not responding to treatment, it is always reasonable to suggest a second opinion, but do not undermine treatment by suggesting that the health worrier should take less medicine than that which was prescribed, or more, or some other medicine in addition.

In short, make sure you do not complicate treatment by interfering with it. A typical board-certified internist has had four years of medical schooling, four years of additional specialized training and a minimum of two years experience dealing with all the intricacies of medical illness. No lay person can pretend to such well-founded judgment.

Do not report to the health-worrier interesting anecdotes of medical catastrophes that have come to your attention. Health worriers are suggestible. They do not need much encouragement to begin wondering whether some rare calamity can happen to them too. Keep in mind that unusual events are just that, unusual. Make that point if you are going to tell such stories. Try not to draw conclusions from random events in the neighborhood. An illness in a neighbor need not strike in your family even if you ate in the same restaurant or slept over in the neighbor's home. If two other neighbors developed leukemia, it does not mean that there is some influence-toxic waste, perhaps, or electromagnetic waves from high-tension wires- that is likely to affect someone in your family. Do not promote these rumors. Outbreaks of illness occur in communities from time to time purely as statistical quirks with no other underlying cause.

Do not repeat health tips (warnings) you heard from your grandmother. These old-wives' tales:

"You'll get cramps if you swim right after eating lunch."

"You'll get sick if you stay up too late studying for an exam."

"You'll get sick if you read too much."

and countless others add up to the conclusion that many ordinary activities endanger health. This is a message that health worriers have already learned only too well.

*   *   *

There are things you can do to help.

Be sympathetic. It may be obvious to you that the health worrier in your family is worrying to an extent way out of proportion to those symptoms he or she has, but it is not obvious to that person. In any case, the distress that person feels is real. Remember, also, that health worriers are not making up imaginary complaints. Their pain, if that is what they are experiencing, although subjective, is real. In most cases they have plainly discernible symptoms which grow out of an ordinary illness of one sort or another. Their problem is primarily that they misinterpret those symptoms and consider them more serious than they really are. They tend to believe that they are much sicker than they really are.

Sympathy is reasonable: constant reassurance is not. It is possible to understand the health worrier's wish for reassurance without giving in to it. Explain that you are not being impatient, but that you know that repeating the same presumably comforting remarks over and over again does not really comfort but only serves to focus still more attention on the possibility of being seriously ill. You will not want to fall in with their habit of examining their bodies for signs of illness; but you should explain that your unwillingness to go along with such a request comes from a wish to help and not from a lack of concern.

Encourage the search for truth. There are a number of kinds of truth important to health worriers. Do the symptoms they have really portend a serious illness or not? Do the drugs they are taking really have a particular side effect or not? Is their illness likely to worsen or not? What, really, are the chances that the particular illness they are worrying about is likely to strike them? If, in fact, they have little to worry about, the facts that they and you discover will support that conclusion.[1]

---

[1] One particular fact, it seems to me, is not worth pursuing. It is not usually possible to find out why exactly someone has become ill at precisely that particular time and not six months or six years earlier or in some time in the future. Usually the reason is too obscure to ferret out and is usually not relevant to proper treatment anyway.

The usual advice to a health worrier-to avoid reading anything upsetting - is wrong and self-defeating. There are very few worries in any area of life, for that matter, that are dispelled by doing nothing. Worrying more - at first - comes inevitably from confronting any fearful subject or circumstance and is the price that must be paid to overcome that fear eventually. Also, the systematic attempt to discover the facts of a possible illness gives health worriers a sense of control over their thoughts. Putting one's hands over the ears, sometimes literally, to block out upsetting news is an unworkable strategy. If you are careful, you, yourself, can try locating information helpful to the health worrier. Stay away from sensational news articles designed more to sell newspapers than to provide accurate information. Remind the health worrier that what he or she reads in the popular press may not be accurate and should be checked against other sources, such as the family doctor.[1]   When a critical consultation with the doctor is looming, it may be a good idea-given the patient's consent-for you to be present. If you are calmer, you may be able to listen more accurately than the health worrier, who tends to get distracted. Doctors often ramble; and health worriers are likely to fix on a casual remark that has no relevance to the doctor's medical opinion about their own particular case. Without meaning to, they listen for the worrisome fact and forget everything else.

Encourage the health worrier to participate in a treatment program such as the one described in these pages. If there is no such program yet organized in your community, this book and Worried Sick? The Workbook can be used as a guide. There is evidence from the cognitive-behavioral treatment of other related disorders that such a home treatment program can work.

[1.] Not, however, about the treatment of health anxiety itself. Too often a doctor's response to the health worrier's concerns is simply "Don't worry," or "Don't read about cancer if you don't have cancer."

Sometimes health worriers do not recognize that they worry too much. The facts of their health seem to them to justify their worrying. More often they know only too well that they have an exaggerated fear of illness but do not see how they can change. No one chooses to worry unnecessarily. When they are in the midst of a particular concern over a particular illness that is threatening them or a member of their family, then they are focused exclusively on that concern and will want to put off treatment of any psychological problem they may have even if they recognize they have such a problem. The rest of the time they do not want to be reminded of their health anxiety. They like to think that this worry is gone forever when the immediate danger is past. More accurately, perhaps, they do not like to think about it at all. So, there is no right time for treatment. Besides, proper treatment is always uncomfortable and, sometimes, downright unpleasant. Sometimes a family member can motivate someone who, for all these reasons, is otherwise disinclined to begin treatment.

In order for treatment to have a reasonable chance of success, it is important to adhere to all parts of the program. Record keeping may not seem to be essential at first glance, but it is. Different records serve different purposes. For example, the health worrier can learn by keeping track which physical symptoms grow out of emotional stress and are less likely, therefore, to be a sign of some other, more serious, disorder. Another example: all the previous times the health worrier turned out to have been wrong in imagining the worst become more and more evident if recorded in a notebook that can be reviewed from time to time. And so, the fundamental Bad Idea of health worriers —that they are really sicker than is apparent— is contradicted by the records.[1] Encourage the health worrier not to choose among those elements of treatment that may seem more or less important to him or to her; they are all important.

[1] For a detailed explanation of record keeping, see Worried Sick? The Workbook.

* * *

Health anxiety is a stubborn problem, likely to recur from time to time whenever the health worrier gets sick or develops a new and not immediately explicable physical complaint. It is a chronic, but not intractable, emotional disorder. The Bad Ideas which underlie health anxiety are long-lasting and difficult to eradicate. For this reason, treatment should be entered into wholeheartedly. Failure leads to cynicism, and subsequent treatment may then become impossible.

Families are affected strongly by any member who is a health worrier. Someone they care about is suffering; and their lives too are disrupted. They get dragged endlessly into reassuring and/or arguing with the health worrier, putting strain on their relationship. Sometimes they, themselves, can become convinced the health worrier is suffering some devastating disease. But there is another reason to encourage that person to overcome this distressing emotional problem: Bad Ideas, like all ideas, are contagious. Health anxiety runs in families. It is desirable that children grow up unafraid and free in particular of the notion that serious illness lurks ominously behind every minor symptom. If parents are health worriers, that attitude is likely to be passed down to their children and often to succeeding generations. Everyone in the family has a stake, therefore, in successfully treating this condition before it can spread.

Chapter Fourteen: A Matter of Perspective

Everyday experience shows that some people are frightened in circumstances where others are not. When someone is very frightened, it often seems to that person that those who are not are foolish and reckless. Those others in turn are likely to regard that person as foolish, or, possibly, neurotic. Someone afraid that the airplane she is sitting in may crash is astonished by all the people sitting next to her reading newspapers or conversing calmly. A man who has ridden a motorcycle every day for the previous ten years cannot understand why there are others who think motorcycles are inherently dangerous. Sometimes these views are strongly felt. One couple living in the northeast lay in a week's supplies of food and candles in case a hurricane should come up suddenly. Their neighbors do not. Each couple considers the other a little crazy. Health worriers, some of them, at least, think it is sensible to worry about diet, germs, medication side effects and a half dozen other things that never enter the thoughts of most people. <u>Whether or not someone worries about a particular danger does not usually depend on an accurate determination of risk</u>. The determining factors are attitudes learned while growing up and the particular circumstances in which one finds oneself as an adult. Well-publicized dangers or dramatic events such as a plane crash make an impression out of proportion to the real risk. Living among frightened people teaches one to be afraid; and whole communities have concluded that the world was about to come to an end the following week.

These beliefs, which are sometimes so poorly supported they might better be called prejudices, are not entirely resistant to change. To an extent they can be countered by contrary evidence, that is, the truth. Even a religious fanatic who expects to die with the rest of the world on Tuesday begins to have second thoughts by the time Wednesday comes around. Moreover, there is an advantage in general in knowing the truth. If some situation is truly dangerous, as can be determined by science or at least by scientific methods of inquiry, it becomes possible to take measures to minimize the risk. If there is truly no danger, it becomes possible finally to put away worrying. To ignore certain risks may be fatal; to worry endlessly about an imaginary danger is tragic. Examples of the former, repeated over and over, are those many people who literally kill themselves because of ignoring the well-publicized dangers of smoking or careless sexual behavior. On some level they do not understand how close they are to dying. Examples of the latter are more likely to go unnoticed.

Theodore came to psychotherapy at the age of 60. He had a lifelong preoccupation with the possibility of dying from a heart attack. At the age of 17 he felt some kind of heart irregularity, just what kind could not be determined from the perspective of 43 years later. He had not gone to a doctor as a youth because he was afraid of what the doctor might tell him. He persisted in avoiding doctors for the next 40 years despite no lessening of his "heart problem." He was depressed much of that time, he said, because he thought that during any moment of excitement his heart was likely to give out. Finally, at the age of 66 he did indeed die from a heart attack.

Theodore turned out to be right in a way. Like very many other people, he was destined to die of a heart attack, but not when he was 17 years old or 27 or 37.

Worrying is what happens in the face of a concern for which there is no clear remedy. One may worry about losing a job in the middle of an economic recession. A common worry is about money especially if a sudden debt such as college tuition looms up. Probably, people worry most about their children since what happens to them is largely out of their control. In order to manage life effectively it is appropriate to be anxious from time to time. This sense of unease drives people to take appropriate measures when confronting a crisis. It is only when there are no measures to take that ordinary anxiety becomes worry. Worry seems pointless only because it comes from the inability to develop a plan for action when such a plan seems necessary.

Theodore worried because he presumed he was in an inescapable danger. He was wrong to think he was in danger and wrong to think there was nothing he could do to avoid that danger even if it had been real. Worrying had become a habit of mind. The truth could have freed him to live more successfully and certainly calmly.

In order to live successfully and calmly, there are certain general truths about life that everyone must accept. In order for a health worrier to stop worrying, that person must come to terms with these facts, some of which are reassuring and some of which are not.

First, during the course of a lifetime everyone will become ill many times unavoidably. Most sicknesses will disappear on their own or with the help of medical treatment. Some become chronic and require continuing medical care to minimize their effect. Except in rare circumstances, these conditions do not seem to prevent people from living busy and happy lives. Life is not ruined by getting sick. Usually. People manage whatever pain and physical impairment they may have without dwelling on them. Usually they think about their illnesses only when they take a turn for the worst.

There are more and more medicines available all the time and more reason to take them. There are drugs being developed now to prevent illnesses in addition to lessening their effects or curing them. Huge amounts of money have been expended to make these drugs safe. And they are safe, not entirely perhaps, but safe enough that most people will never have a serious drug reaction.

People are living longer all the time. The chance of dying prematurely is dropping and has been dropping steadily over the last century. Similarly, the effects of different illnesses, and accidents too, have been lessened by continuing technological innovations. As a consequence, the physical quality of life is getting better for older people. Surgery is being performed reasonably on older and older patients. Whether or not someone is truly old when he or she reaches the age of 70, or thereabouts depends on attitudes and other factors not necessarily tied to age per se.

There are people in their seventies who work at something, perhaps not their original occupation but at something they consider interesting and worthwhile, taking care of grandchildren, perhaps, instead of children. They still take pleasure in seeing friends. Their most intimate relationships have not paled. They are physically active. The social activities and forms of entertainment that have always meant something to them still do. If they have been active politically or in their church, they are still. They participate in things. They look forward to making new friends and visiting places new to them. They are still curious. They are still learning. With the exception of having more children, everything they ever aspired to is still within reach. They are still treated with respect by others. Such a person is not old. He, or she, may well be coping with a chronic disease such as diabetes or arthritis, but it has not made life unsatisfying. Very many people report this to be the happiest time of their lives.

Conversely, someone who has nothing to do all day long, who has no hopes for the future, and who takes no pleasure in the ordinary commerce of life is old and may have become old in middle age. It is the ways people live throughout their lives that determine how well they manage the last part of life.

If being old is defined by attitude, being very old is defined by circumstances. Inevitably, sooner or later, as a consequence simply of not dying, the very old must endure the death of friends, of a spouse, and, sometimes, even of children. Illnesses multiply. Work becomes impossible. The increasing loss of hearing and vision serve to isolate the very old. Reading, which may have been a great source of pleasure, becomes difficult or impossible. Even the task of eating and going to the bathroom becomes difficult to manage. Sleep comes on intermittently and at the wrong times. Various pains accumulate, making simple activities like walking hard to do without assistance. Even the very independent are reduced at last to relying on others, often strangers, to take care of them. Often the last acts of life are played out on a set of two rooms, a bedroom and a bathroom. Worst of all, intellectual faculties falter. Memory and concentration are impaired progressively, and in the worst cases the very old forget everything. They forget their families, they forget who they are, and finally they forget how to speak. Anyone who would invest time and energy guarding health in order to reach this extreme old age would be making a bad bargain.

Of course, health worriers are not anxious to live as long as they can. They are afraid of getting old, as they are afraid of dying. They just do not want to die now. It is interesting, therefore, to note that paradoxically, or perhaps not so paradoxically, the older people get and the closer they get to dying, the less they worry about dying! Certainly, someone in the life-long habit of worrying about health or anything else will likely continue to worry into old age, but the fear of death recedes. The great majority of our patients are young people. What accounts for this change of perspective? It is because the value of life changes.

The value of life

One customarily speaks of life being precious - equally precious to everyone; but it is not so. Taking the life of another human being is considered everywhere to be a heinous crime; but the punishment for infanticide in many countries is less that that for the murder of an adult. Many would object vehemently to that idea. It is not that way, or, at least, ought not to be that way, they assert. They understand that in times past people were killed just because they were mentally retarded. Deformed children were abandoned on a hillside to die. In some cultures the vary old or very sick were left somewhere to starve to death. But these were barbarian practices contrary to every ethical principle and every religious belief - at least, current religious belief. Some people go further and believe the sanctity of life begins with conception. Here there is no consensus. Others think life really begins with the implantation of the embryo in the uterus since very many embryos never implant. Certain religious practices suggest life begins at quickening, around the fifth month of pregnancy, when the fetus can be felt to move. Other people, of course, consider life to begin at birth.

Similarly, there are some who consider life to be sacred and should never be purposely ended, even when an individual has been unconscious for years, or in intractable pain, and even when that individual is expressing the wish to die. Others think it is ethical to cause such an individual to die. These beliefs are controversial now. Even in situations where it might seem obvious to one person that life is no longer worth living, there are others who will disagree. Many people mourn terribly the loss of an abnormal pregnancy, when others would not. Some would mourn similarly over the death of an aged parent who had faded away years before because of Alzheimer's disease. Particular deaths may be very painful. On the other hand, how often do people say: "It is good that mom (or dad) died now without suffering longer?" They judge their parents' life to have lost its value.

The right to life, however it may be defined, is and ought to be explicit in our constitution and in the laws of every civilized society. Nevertheless, however equal everyone may be under the law, society makes the uncomfortable judgment that some lives are worth more than others. Men in the secret service are trained to sacrifice themselves, if necessary, to save the life of the President. The effects of a presidential assassination are so dire that most people see this as appropriate. Policemen and firemen, and soldiers too, routinely risk their lives to save others; and there are times when they knowingly give up their lives to do so. Ordinary people make similar sacrifices. The fact is that people's lives are valued differently in our culture depending on a number of circumstances. <u>Similarly, the value some-one places on his or her own life changes over time in a way consis-</u>

tent with these societal views. Almost always, elderly parents would sacrifice their lives for their children, and some have done so. Those adult children might very well sacrifice their lives for their own children, but not for their parents. The death of a young parent is more tragic than the death of an old man or an infant. Drawn in such stark terms, a person's life may be said to be more valuable at certain stages of life than at others.

Three overlapping factors determine just how valuable is someone's life:

1. <u>How much longer that person might reasonably be expected to live.</u> A 70 year old man told that his cancer might return 10 years later worried very little because he thought he might not live another 10 years in any case. When he was 30 he had worried much more over medical problems that were much less severe.

2. <u>How much responsibility that person may have.</u> A health worrier who worries about dying primarily because she thinks her orphaned children could not manage without her has no reason to worry any longer if her children are now adults with children of their own. In general, the arc of responsibility is highest at a time of first becoming a parent. The death through accident or violence of such a person is especially poignant because the role he or she plays is so important. On the other hand, someone who is elderly and who no longer works, or is unable to work, counts himself, or herself, as less important. And society in general agrees. Yet it is this shrinking responsibility that frees older people to do other things and accounts in part for their being happy. <u>The possibility of dying calls up fewer regrets for the aged because what they do is less critical</u>.

3. <u>How good or how bad is the quality of that person's life?</u> Life is precious to someone who is enjoying it. At the other extreme are those who are disabled or in intractable pain. As

264

in the case of those who are clinically depressed, someone can feel so miserable and so hopeless that life takes on a negative value, and suicide seems preferable to continued struggle. The tragedy of suicide is that only a few weeks after taking medicine the perspective of the depressed person can change radically. As time goes on, though, and old people become very old and are often lonely and unhappy in myriad other ways, they speak of it being "time to go." Usually they confront their impending death without bitterness and with equanimity. Thinking back on their lives, as they often do, they are content. <u>Dying is less awful for the aged because there is less satisfaction in living</u>.

And then, in the end, everyone does die. The meaning of life - the purpose of life - cannot be sought in permanent things. People do not last. The things they accomplish in life do not last forever. Over the span of hundreds of years everyone is forgotten. People cannot be committed simply to living as long as possible. The meaning of life has to be found in the things people do every day. Life may be a struggle, but plainly most people enjoy it. Most people are happy most of the time. Besides the ordinary physical pleasures familiar to everyone - walking about on a pleasant day, listening to music, looking at a painting, dancing - there are those activities that tie us to other people. Human beings are social animals. What matters most are family, friends, and the larger human community, of which we are a part. Therein lies most of life's pleasures. The extraordinary grip of our ties to other people cannot be explained except to say that it is inherent in the kind of creature we are. The day we make someone else laugh, or help someone up who has fallen, or teach something to somebody, is a good day. A day spent worrying over some imaginary danger to no purpose is a wasted day. Too many wasted days can spoil life altogether.

Most people do not worry about dying because death seems remote. But there are many people who do not seem troubled even in the face of imminent death. A famous example is Socrates, whose last thoughts before dying were not of escaping a death sentence, which he could have done, but of repaying a small debt which he owed. He was calm and scolded his friends who had gathered around for not being calm also. The term "gallows humor" refers to the very real phenomenon of the condemned making jokes just before a noose is slipped around their neck. Many people die without warning and without having to think about the process of dying, but those who die slowly over a period of time usually enter a stage of acceptance where they are not worried about dying. They worry instead about the effect of their illness and death on their families or about some unfinished and important work. They are more the rule than the exception. What allows these people to face death with equanimity? Is there a lesson here for health worriers?

This chapter is a recommendation to health worriers and, for that matter, to others who are caught up day after day with particular concerns, whether it is making money, or climbing up a corporate ladder, or driving one's children to do a little better academically than their neighbor's children, to step back for a moment and consider what is really important. Not uncommonly, those who have suffered a heart attack say it was the best thing that ever happened to them. Instead of being driven by what seems now to be a pointless struggle to do something that turned out not to be doable at all, they had the chance to rethink their lives and reorder their priorities.

This book presents a program to lessen the irrational fears of health anxiety. It is a way of coming truly to know about health and illness so that worrying for no good reason can be put away. But between the efforts to ward off disease and other efforts to ward off the worry about disease, there is time to stop for a little while to think about a larger purpose. It should not be necessary to grow old to grow wise.

Those people who are not concerned about dying have not stopped caring about everything; they care very much about some things, more than life itself. Socrates thought of himself as an honest man, willing to speak the truth whatever the consequences and unafraid of the disapproval of others. If he were to have run away, he would have given up something more important to him that his life; he would have been untrue to the person he had always striven to be. Those who laugh at their executioners are making a statement; you can kill me, but you cannot make me cower. In laughing, they achieve a kind of victory over death. Many ordinary people are determined to maintain their dignity in the face of death. They know they would be upsetting their family and friends, and embarrassing themselves, were they to slide into hysterics or shake their fist at God. But the truth is they do not feel hysterical. Most people relax when they know once and for all what will happen to them. They are not inclined to rail against the absurdities of life-that nothing we struggle to do lasts, that life itself does not last. Like all animals, we have built in the wish to survive, but unlike other animals, we know we cannot. With the end of struggle in view there is acceptance and peace. Usually.

This, then, is the lesson to learn. A medical crisis, like any crisis, allows for change. It is a time to stand back from the ordinary preoccupations of life that take up so much time and energy and decide what really matters. Every person has an idea of himself, or herself, that is worth living up to, or sometimes, dying for. "I am worthwhile" each person must be able to say, "because I do these particular things that are worthwhile. I have accomplished this much in my work. I have had a good effect on people. They can count on me to help them and care about them. I am a good parent. I always try my best. I am reliable. I have tried to protect myself and the people I care for. I have made a difference in the lives of other people. I stand for this. I am committed. This is who I am. Whatever happens to me tomorrow, even if I should get sick and die, these things still count. Whether I live or die matters less because these other things matter more."

No one can be indifferent to the prospect of dying. The pain of dying is shared by anyone close to the dying person and for that reason alone cannot be dismissed by any trick of the mind. But it is possible for someone who is relatively young and vigorous to do what someone who is close to death usually does, that is, to take stock. Illness, even serious illness, occurs from time to time. It is part of the human condition. The rest of life must not be given over to lamenting this fact. If health worriers can find meaning in who they are and in what they do, it is possible with that new perspective to live sensibly and joyfully.

The Anxiety & Phobia Center
White Plains Hospital Center

Chief Complaint _____

Tentative Diagnosis _____

HEALTH ANXIETY SCALE

	Yes	No
Do you feel that you are likely to get sick more frequently than others, or are likely to get sicker than others when you do get sick?		
Do you think a lot about the possibility of getting illnesses that run in your family?		
When you develop physical symptoms, do you immediately contemplate the most serious illness that could explain these symptoms?		
Do you often think how terrible it would be for you or your children if you were to die prematurely?		
Are you under the impression that it is very important to get to a doctor at the first sign of getting sick?		
Do you visit doctors much more frequently than you really need to in order to be reassured about your health?		
Do you avoid doctors because you are frightened about what they might discover?		
Do you leave the doctor's office sometimes unsure of what he said or meant because you were nervous when he spoke to you?		
Although you know medical opinions can never be certain, do you nevertheless ask your doctor questions such as "are you sure I don't have ... cancer ... or AIDS ... or high blood pressure, etc.?" Is it hard for the doctor to reassure you?		
Do you ask what the cause of a symptom is even when the doctor has told you that that symptom is inconsequential?		

Do you ask your doctor to do medical tests in order "to be sure" even if the doctor is not otherwise inclined to order such tests?		
Do you worry for days ahead of time about routine tests such as a mammogram?		
Do you worry when a laboratory test result falls outside the normal range?		
Do you hesitate to take prescribed medicines because of concern about side effects?		
Are you more sensitive to medication than other people?		
Are you more inclined to take "natural" substances, such as herbs, rather than prescribed medicines?		
Do you worry when you have trouble sleeping or if your bowels are irregular?		
Do you check parts of your body over and over again looking for an abnormality such as a lump?		
Do you often suffer palpitations?		
Do you ask other people, such as a spouse, whether you are looking a little better today or a little worse?		
Do you worry about germs or about catching someone else's illness?		
Do you worry about very unlikely diseases such as a brain aneurysm that tend to lurk silently and may suddenly kill you?		
Are you preoccupied much of the time with thoughts of becoming ill or dying to the point, sometimes, where family members feel obligated to reassure you?		
Do you feel your health worries are foolish?		

THE ANXIETY & PHOBIA TREATMENT CENTER
HEALTH ANXIETY PROGRAM

How many times a day does a health worry occur to you? _____

Do your health worries interfere with your life?

They spoil much of my life   _____

They interfere a great deal   _____

They interfere to a moderate degree   _____

They interfere somewhat   _____

They interfere not at all   _____

Name_____ Date _____

Diagnostic Criteria of the Diagnostic and Statistical Manual (IV) of the American Psychiatric Association

Hypochondriasis

A. Preoccupation with fears of having or the idea that one has a serious disease based on the person's misinterpretation of bodily symptoms.

B. The preoccupation persists despite appropriate medical evaluation and reassurance.

C. The belief in Criterion A is not of delusional intensity (as in Delusional Disorder, Somatic Type) and is not restricted to a circumscribed concern about appearance (as in Body Dysmorphic Disorder).

D. The preoccupation causes clinically significant distress or impairment in social, occupational or other important areas of functioning.

E. The duration of the disturbance is at least 6 months.

F. The preoccupation is not better accounted for by Generalized Anxiety Disorder. Obsessive-Compulsive Disorder, Panic Disorder, a Major Depressive Episode, Separation Anxiety, or another Somatoform Disorder.

Specify if

With Poor Insight: if, for most of the time during the current episode, the person does not recognize that the concern about having a serious illness is excessive or unreasonable.

Somatization Disorder

A. A history of many physical complaints beginning before age 30 years that occur over a period of several years and result in treatment being sought or significant impairment in social occupational, or other important areas of functioning.

B. Each of the following criteria must have been met, with individual symptoms occurring at any time during the course of the disturbance.

1) <u>Four pain symptoms</u>: a history of pain related to at least four different sites or functions (e.g., head, abdomen, back, joints, extremities, chest, and rectum. During menstruation, during sexual intercourse, or during urination).

2) <u>Two gastrointestinal</u> symptoms: a history of at least two gastrointestinal symptoms other than pain (e.g. nausea, bloating, vomiting other than during pregnancy, diarrhea, or intolerance of several different foods).

3) <u>One sexual symptom</u>: a history of at least one sexual or reproductive symptom other than pain (e.g. sexual indifference, erectile or ejaculatory dysfunction, irregular menses, excessive menstrual bleeding, vomiting throughout pregnancy).

4) <u>One psudoneurological symptom:</u> a history of at least one symptom or deficit suggesting a neurological condition not limited to pain (conversion symptoms such as impaired coordination or balance, paralysis or localized weakness, difficulty swallowing or lump in throat, aphonia, urinary retention, hallucinations, loss of touch or pain sensation, double vision, blindness, deafness, seizures, dissociative symptoms such as amnesia, or loss of consciousness other than fainting)

C. Either (1) or (2)

1. After appropriate investigation, each of the symptoms in Criterion B cannot be fully explained by a known general medical condition or the direct effects of a substance (e.g. drug of abuse, a medication).

2. When there is a related general medical condition the physical complaints or resulting social or occupational impairment are in excess of what would be expected from the history, physical examination or laboratory findings.

D. The symptoms are not intentionally produced or feigned (as in Factitious Disorder or Malingering).

Panic

A discrete period of intense fear or discomfort, in which four (or more) of the following symptoms developed abruptly and reached a peak within 10 minutes.

1. Palpitations, pounding heart, or accelerated heart rate
2. Sweating
3. Trembling or shaking
4. Sensations of shortness of breath or smothering
5. Feeling of choking
6. Chest pain or discomfort
7. Nausea or abdominal distress
8. Feeling dizzy, unsteady, lighthearted, or faint
9. Derealization (feelings of unreality) or depersonalization (being detached from oneself)
10. Fear of losing control or going crazy
11. Fear of dying
12. Paresthesias (numbness or tingling sensations)
13. Chills or hot flashes

Obsessive-Compulsive Disorder

A. Either obsession or compulsions

Obsessions as defined by (1), (2), (3) and (4)

1. Recurrent and persistent thoughts, impulses or images that are experienced at some time during the disturbance, as intrusive and inappropriate and that cause marked anxiety or distress

2. The thoughts, impulses, or images are not simply excessive worries about real-life problems

3. The person attempts to ignore or suppress such thoughts, impulses, or images or to neutralize them with some other thought or action.

4. The person recognizes that the obsessional thoughts, impulses, or images are a product of his or her own mind (not imposed from without as in thought insertion).

Compulsions as defined by (1) and (2):

1. Repetitive behaviors (e.g., hand washing, ordering, checking) or mental acts (e.g. praying, counting, repeating words silently) that the person feels driven to perform in response to an obsession, or according to rules that must be applied rigidly.

2. The behaviors or mental acts are aimed at preventing or reducing distress or preventing some dreaded event or situation; however, these behaviors or mental acts either are not connected in a realistic way with what they are designed to neutralize or prevent or are clearly excessive.

B. At some point during the course of the disorder, the person has recognized that the obsessions or compulsions are excessive or unreasonable. **Note:** this does not apply to children.

C. The obsessions or compulsions cause marked distress, are time consuming (take more than I hour a day), or significantly interfere with the person's normal routine occupational (or academic) functioning, or usual social activities or relationships.

D. If another Axis I disorder is present, the content of the obsessions or compulsions is not restricted to it (e.g. preoccupation with food in the presence of an Eating Disorder, hair pulling in the presence of Trichotillomania: concern with appearance in the presence of Body Dysmorphic Disorder: preoccupation with drugs in the presence of a Substance Use Disorder: preoccupation with having a serious illness in the presence of Hypochondriasis: preoccupation with sexual urges or fantasies in the presence of a Paraphilia: or guilty ruminations in the presence of Major Depression Disorders).

E. The disturbance is not due to the direct physiological effects of a substance (e.g., a drug of abuse, a medication) or a general medical condition.

Major Depressive Episode

A. Five (or more) of the following symptoms have been present during the same 2 week period and represent a change from previous functioning, at least one of the symptoms is either (1) depressed mood or (2) loss of interest or pleasure.

Note: Do not include symptoms that are clearly due to a general medical condition, or mood-incongruent delusions or hallucinations.

1. Depressed mood most of the day, nearly every day, as indicated by either subjective report (e.g. feels sad or empty) or observation made by others (e.g., appears tearful). **Note:** in children and adolescents, can be irritable mood.

2. Markedly diminished interest or pleasure in all, or almost all, activities most of the day, nearly every day (as indicated by either subjective account or observation made by others).

3 . Significant weight loss when not dieting or weight gain (e.g. a change of more than 5 % of body weight in a month), or decrease or increase in appetite nearly every day. **Note:** in children consider failure to make expected weight gains.

4. Insomnia or hypersomnia nearly every day.

5. Psychomotor agitation or retardation nearly every day (observable by others, not merely subjective feelings of restlessness or being slowed down).

6. Fatigue or loss of energy nearly every day.

7. Feelings of worthlessness or excessive or inappropriate guilt (which may be delusional) nearly every day (not merely self-reproach or guilt about being sick).

8. Diminished ability to think or concentrate, or indecisiveness, nearly every day (either by subjective account or as observed by others).

9. Recurrent thoughts of death (not just fear of dying), recurrent suicidal ideation without a specific plan or a suicide attempt or a specific plan for committing suicide.

B. The symptoms do not meet criteria for a Mixed Episode.

C. The symptoms cause clinically significant distress or impairment in social, occupational, or other important areas of functioning.

D. The symptoms are not due to the direct physiological effects of a substance (e.g., a drug of abuse, a medication) or a general medical condition (e.g., hypothyroidism).

E. The symptoms are not better accounted for by Bereavement, i.e., after the loss of a loved one, the symptoms persist for longer than 2 months or are characterized by marked functional impairment, morbid preoccupation with worthlessness, suicidal ideation, psychotic symptoms, or psychomotor retardation.

Generalized Anxiety Disorder
(Includes Overanxious Disorder of Childhood)

A. Excessive anxiety and worry (apprehensive expectation), occurring more days that not for at least 6 months, about a number of events or activities (such as work or school performance).

B. The person finds it difficult to control the worry.

C. The anxiety and worry are associated with three (or more) of the following six symptoms (with at least some symptoms present for more days than not for the past 6 months) **Note:** Only one item is required in children

   1. Restlessness or feeling keyed up or on edge
   2. Being easily fatigued
   3. Difficulty concentrating or mind going blank
   4. Irritability
   5. Muscle tension
   6. Sleep disturbance (difficulty falling or staying asleep, or restless unsatisfying sleep)

D. The focus of the anxiety and worry is not confined to features of an Axis I disorder e.g., the anxiety or worry is not about having a Panic Attack (as in Panic Disorder) being embarrassed in public (as in Social Phobia), being contaminated (as in Obsessive-Compulsive Disorder), being away from home or close relatives (as in Separation Anxiety Disorder), gaining weight (as in Anorexia Nervosa), having multiple physical complaints (as in Somatization Disorder), or having a serious illness (as in Hypochondriasis) and the anxiety and worry do not occur exclusively during Posttraumatic Stress Disorder.

E. The anxiety, worry, or physical symptoms cause clinically significant distress or impairment in social, occupational, or other important areas of functioning.

F. The disturbance is not due to the direct physiological effects of a substance (e.g. a drug of abuse, a medication) or a general medical condition (e.g., hyperthyroidism) and does not occur exclusively during a Mood Disorder, a Psychotic Disorder, or a Pervasive Developmental Disorder.

Lightning Source UK Ltd.
Milton Keynes UK
UKHW030613211220
375566UK00004B/258